O O L
OXFORD ONCOLOGY LIBRARY

JAN 2013

Colorectal Cancer

Oxford University Press makes no representation, express or implied, that the drug dosages in this book are correct. Readers must therefore always check the product information and clinical procedures with the most up-to-date published product information and data sheets provided by the manufacturers and the most recent codes of conduct and safety regulations. The authors and the publishers do not accept responsibility or legal liability for any errors in the text or for the misuse or misapplication of material in this work.

▶ Except where otherwise stated, drug doses and recommendations are for the non-pregnant adult who is not breast-feeding.

O O L
OXFORD ONCOLOGY LIBRARY

Colorectal Cancer

Edited by

Daniel Swinson

Consultant and Honorary Senior Lecturer in
GI Medical Oncology,
St James's Institute of Oncology,
University of Leeds,
Leeds, UK

Matthew Seymour

Cancer Research UK Cancer Medicine Research Unit,
St James's Institute of Oncology,
University of Leeds,
Leeds, UK

OXFORD
UNIVERSITY PRESS

OXFORD
UNIVERSITY PRESS

Great Clarendon Street, Oxford OX2 6DP,
United Kingdom

Oxford University Press is a department of the University of Oxford.
It furthers the University's objective of excellence in research, scholarship,
and education by publishing worldwide. Oxford is a registered trade mark of
Oxford University Press in the UK and in certain other countries

British Library Cataloguing in Publication Data

Data available

Library of Congress Cataloging in Publication Data

Data available

ISBN 978–0–19–959020–9

Printed in Great Britain
on acid-free paper by
Ashford Colour Press Ltd., Gosport, Hampshire

Contents

Contributors

Robert A. Adair
Dept of Hepatobiliary &
Transplant Surgery,
St James's University Hospital,
Leeds, UK

Alan Anthoney
Institute of Oncology,
St James's Hospital, Leeds, UK

Mike Braun
The Christie NHS Foundation
Trust, Manchester,
Greater Manchester, UK

Fiona Collinson
Institute of Oncology,
St James's Hospital, Leeds, UK

Rachel Cooper
Institute of Oncology,
St James's Hospital, Leeds, UK

Luis Daverede
Institute of Oncology,
St James's University Hospital,
Leeds, UK

David R. Ferry
Royal Wolverhampton
Hospitals Trust, UK

Peter Hall
Institute of Oncology,
St James's Hospital, Leeds, UK

Paul Hatfield
Institute of Oncology,
St James's Hospital, Leeds, UK

Uschi Hofmann
Huddersfield Royal Infirmary,
Lindley, Huddersfield, UK

Bill Hulme
Prince Of Wales Hospice,
Pontefract, UK

Zahirul Huq
Consultant Colorectal Surgeon
Department of Colorectal
Surgery
North Manchester General
Hospital
Manchester, UK

Kai J. Leong
Department of Academic
Surgery
University Hospitals
Birmingham NHS Foundation
Trust, Birmingham, UK

Christopher Macklin
Dewsbury Hospital, Mid-Yorks
NHS Trust, Yorkshire, UK

Ian S. Morgan
Royal Wolverhampton
Hospitals Trust, UK

Dion Morton
Queen Elizabeth Hospital,
Birmingham, UK

Christopher Ramsey
Leeds Teaching Hospitlas
Leeds, UK

Peter M. Sagar
Institute of Oncology,
St James's Hospital, Leeds, UK

Dominic Slade
Salford Royal NHS Foundation
Trust, Salford, Greater
Manchester, UK

CONTRIBUTORS

Daniel Swinson
Institute of Oncology,
St James's Hospital, Leeds, UK

Giles J. Toogood
Dept of Hepatobiliary &
Transplant Surgery, St James's
University Hospital, Leeds, UK

Harpreet Wasan
Imperial College Healthcare
NHS Trust, London, UK

Alastair L. Young
Dept of Hepatobiliary &
Transplant Surgery, St James's
University Hospital, Leeds, UK

Abbreviations

AFAP	attenuated FAP
AHPBA	American Hepato-Pancreato-Biliary Association
APC	adenomatosis polyposis coli
APC	antigen presenting cells
APER	abdomino-perineal excision of rectum
APR	abdomino-perineal resection
BED	biologically effective doses
BSC	best supportive care
CEA	carcinoembryonic antigen
CHRPE	congenital hypertrophy of the retinal pigment epithelium
CIN	chromosomal instability
CRC	colorectal cancer
CRLM	colorectal liver metastasis
CRM	circumferential resection margin
CT	computed tomography
CTC	CT colonography
DC	dendritic cells
DFI	disease free interval
dG	de Gramont
DOM	tolerance-breaking domain
DPD	dihydropyrimidine dehydrogenase
DTH	delayed-type hypersensitivity
EBUS	endobronchial ultrasound
EGFR	epidermal growth factor receptor
EMVI	extra-mural vascular invasion
EPIC	European Prospective Investigation into Cancer and Nutrition
EPOC	Eloxatin® for peri-operative use
ERUS	endo-rectal ultrasound
EUS	endoscopic ultrasound
FAP	familial adenomatous polyposis
FBAL	fluoro-β-alanine

FDG-PET	flourodeoxyglucose positron emission tomography
FLOX	5FU/Leucovorin/Oxaliplatin
FOLFOX	5FU/Leucovorin and Oxaliplatin
FNCLCC	Federation Nationale des Centres de Lutte Contre le Cancer
G-FOBT	guaiac-based test
GWA	Genome Wide Association
HA	hepatic arterial
HER	human epidermal growth factor receptor
HNPCC	hereditary non-polyposis colon cancer
HRT	hormone replacement therapy
HSP	anti-heat shock proteins
I-FOBT	immunochemical-based tests
IGRT	image-guided radiation therapy
IHC	immunohistochemistry
IMRT	intensity modulated radiotherapy
INT US	Intergroup
JP	juvenile polyposis
JPS	juvenile polyposis syndrome
KRAS	Kirsten rat sarcoma
LOH	loss of heterozgosity
LS	Lynch syndrome
LV	leucovorin
MALDI-TOF	Matrix Assisted Laser Desorption Ionization–Time of Flight
MAP	MYH associated polyposis
MdG	modified de Gramont
MDT	multidisciplinary team
MMR	mismatch repair
MRI	magnetic resonance imaging
MSI	microsatellite instability
MSS	microsatellite stable
MUT	mutation
MVA	modified vaccinia Ankara
MYH	MutY homologue
NICE	National Institute for Health and Clinical Excellence
NSAID	non-steroidal anti-inflammatory analgesics
OS	overall survival

PET	positron emission tomography
PJS	Peutz Jeghers syndrome
PMCC	pulmonary metastasectomy for colorectal cancer
PRR	pattern recognition receptors
PTT	Protein Truncating Test
QALY	quality adjusted life-year
QUASAR	Quick And Simple And Reliable
RCT	randomized controlled trials
RE	radio-embolization
RILD	radiation induced liver disease
R0	resection
RPMI	Roswell Park Memorial institue
RR	response rates
SCPRT	short-course pre-operative radiotherapy
SELDI-TOF	Surface-Enhanced Laser Desorption/Ionization Time-Of-Flight
SIRT	selective internal radiotherapy
SOS	sinusoidal obstructive syndrome
SPS	sphincter preserving surgery
SSAT	Society for Surgery of Alimentary Tract
SSO	Society of Surgical Oncology
TAA	tumour associated antigens
TEMS	transanal endoscopic microsurgery
TME	total mesorectal excision
TP	thymidine phosphylase
TTP	time to disease progression
UC	ulcerative colitis
VATS	video-assisted thoracoscopic surgery
VEGF	vascular endothelial growth factor
VIP	anti-vasoactive intestinal peptide

Chapter 1

Introduction to colorectal cancer

Mike Braun

Key points

- Colorectal cancer (CRC) is one of the three most common incident cancers and causes of cancer related death
- Most CRC is sporadic with approximately 5% of colorectal cancer due to autosomal dominant hereditary conditions (FAP and Lynch syndrome)
- Environmental and dietary factors are important in the development of CRC as evidenced by data from migrant studies. The precise impact of lifestyle factors is difficult to measure due to problems in assessment and consideration of potential confounding factors
- The molecular basis of hereditary and sporadic colorectal cancers is increasingly well understood. Mutations and deletions in key genes such as APC in FAP and the MMR genes in Lynch syndrome have been identified. The step-wise accumulation of genetic abnormalities (*APC, KRAS, p53*, etc) has been recognized in sporadic tumours
- The predominant staging systems are Dukes' and TNM which are used internationally and provide important prognostic information which can guide therapeutic decisions.

1.1 Epidemiology

Globally over one million new cases of colorectal cancer (CRC) were diagnosed worldwide in 2002. In the UK, CRC is diagnosed in over 37,000 people per year and results in over 16,000 deaths per year making it one of the three most common incident cancers and causes of cancer related death. The incidence of colorectal cancer increases with age and over 80% of cases occur over age 60 years. The UK incidence of CRC has remained stable over the last decade and CRC related mortality has significantly reduced since the 1970s.

1.2 Histology

Adenocarcinomas constitute over 95% of colorectal tumours with mucinous, signet ring and medullary histological subtypes defined. Signet ring cell tumours constitute approximately 1% of all CRC. Medullary carcinoma was added to the World Health Organization classification in 2000, and has a characteristic phenotype of non-gland forming carcinoma, right sided location and the presence of tumour infiltrating lymphocytes. Mucinous histology, defined by greater than 50% of the tumour being composed of extracellular mucin, is seen in 10–15%. Mucinous histology, the presence of microsatellite instability, and features of medullary carcinoma have been associated with CRC seen in the hereditary Lynch syndrome.

Rare tumour sub-types such as neuroendocrine tumours (low-grade and high-grade/small cell), lymphomas, squamous cell carcinoma, sarcomas and GI stromal tumours constitute 2–3% of tumours in the colon and rectum. Squamous and neuroendocrine tumours are most commonly found in the rectum whereas the other sub-types are more commonly found in the colon. Outcome data relative to adenocarcinomas is limited but analysis of the United States SEER (Surveillance, Epidemiology, and End Results) national cancer registry between 1991 and 2000 provides useful population-based data. Signet ring carcinomas and small cell carcinomas had a poor prognosis whereas well-differentiated neuroendocrine cancers had a good prognosis.

1.3 Aetiology of colorectal cancer

1.3.1 Acquired factors
1.3.1.1 Geographical variation
There is at least a 25-fold variation in global CRC incidence. The highest incidence rates are seen in developed nations (e.g. North America, Western Europe, Australia, and New Zealand) whereas low incidence rates are seen in many African, Asian, and South American countries. The incidence of CRC in migrants, moving from a low- to a high-risk population shows a rapid increase, and therefore much of this variation is thought to be due to environmental and lifestyle factors. Many CRC low-risk countries have seen significant increases in risk over the last 50 years, which may reflect changes in diet and lifestyle.

Dramatic increases in the CRC risk have been seen in Japan, historically a low incidence area, which in the 1970s and 1980s saw the incidence increase to reach those seen in US Caucasians.

1.3.1.2 Dietary factors

The European Prospective Investigation into Cancer and Nutrition (EPIC) study investigated relationships between diet, lifestyle, genetic and environmental factors, and the incidence of different cancers. Significant associations between CRC risk and increasing intake of red and processed meat (HR 1.57 (95% CI 1.13–2.17)), and a protective effect from eating fish (HR 0.69 (95% CI 0.54–0.88)) and dietary fibre (HR 0.75 (95% CI 0.59–0.95)) were noted. Other studies and a meta-analysis support the association between red and processed meat and CRC risk. Confounding associations between dietary and lifestyle factors are a hazard of association studies. Recent data from EPIC has suggested that fruit and vegetable intake may be protective and reduce colon cancer risk although previous studies have not suggested a strong association. Similarly an inverse relationship between dietary folate intake and CRC risk has been noted. Low dietary fat intake has not been strongly associated with CRC risk.

1.3.1.3 Lifestyle

An increased risk of colorectal cancer has been associated with alcohol consumption and obesity. Alcohol consumption of 30–45g/day (equivalent to two to three alcoholic drinks per day) increases CRC risk by 16% and consumption of >45g/day is associated with 41% increase in risk. Obesity has also been found to increase the risk of colorectal cancer with a dose response relationship observed. In contrast high levels of physical activity over long time periods have been associated with a reduced risk of colorectal cancer. It is uncertain whether tobacco smoking increases CRC risk, although it may negate the benefits of increased fruit and vegetable intake.

1.3.1.4 Other factors

Ulcerative Colitis (UC) has been associated with an increased risk of developing CRC which appears to be associated with the timing of onset (childhood vs. adult) and duration of active colitis. A variety of drugs including non-steroidal anti-inflammatory analgesics (NSAIDs) and hormone replacement therapy (HRT) have been associated with a reduced risk of CRC. Randomized trials have assessed low dose aspirin in patients who had previously had colorectal adenomas, or cancers and reduced the risk of developing colorectal adenomas. However, cohort studies have suggested that significant reductions in CRC risk are only seen after prolonged exposure (>10 years) to aspirin doses higher than are used in cardiovascular disease and which are associated with an increased risk of GI bleeding. The use of aspirin or other NSAIDS for chemo-prevention is not currently advocated.

1.4 **Hereditary colorectal cancer**

A familial risk can be identified in up to 30% of CRC cases but high penetrance hereditary syndromes are identified in up to approximately 5%. Familial Adenomatous Polyposis (FAP) and Lynch syndrome are the two major hereditary conditions, although other rare syndromes have been identified (e.g. MYH, Juvenile Polyposis, Peutz-Jeghers).

1.5 **Familial Adenomatous Polyposis (FAP)**

FAP is an autosomal dominant condition affecting 1 in 13,500 members of the general population, which is defined by the presence of greater than 100 adenomatous polyps within the large bowel although thousands of polyps may be present. There is almost a 100% risk of developing CRC by the 3rd to 5th decades of life. The incidence of FAP related CRC has fallen as family screening programmes have become widespread, and FAP now accounts for less than 0.1% of incident colorectal cancers.

Management of FAP is by screening for polyps and prophylactic colectomy. UK guidelines advise that patients known to carry a mutation should have prophylactic surgery aged 16–20 years. Patients wishing to defer surgery should be counselled regarding CRC risk and undergo intensive colonic surveillance with surgery before age 25 recommended. Families with a history consistent with classical FAP, but no APC mutation identified, should be screened with annual flexible sigmoidoscopy performed from age 13–15 until age 30, and then 3 yearly until age 60.

Extra-colonic manifestations of FAP are frequently seen. Congenital hypertrophy of the retinal pigment epithelium (CHRPE) occurs in approximately 60% of FAP patients. It has no malignant potential but its presence can identify at-risk family members before the develop- ment of colorectal polyps. Desmoid tumours are seen in 10–15% of patients, often in the abdominal wall or cavity, and enlarging des- moid tumours may cause pain or compression of adjacent structures. Gardner's syndrome describes a variant of FAP with the desmoid tumours, epidermoid skin cysts and osteomas. Duodenal disease has become a major cause of morbidity and mortality as the outcome of FAP patients has improved. Duodenal polyposis is seen in up to 65% of FAP patients, and there is a 4% lifetime risk of developing duodenal/peri-ampullary cancer. Upper GI endoscopy every 3 years from age 30 has been advised to screen for duodenal polyposis. Other rare manifestations include cerebellar medulloblastomas (Turcot's syndrome), Papillary carcinoma of the thyroid, and adrenocortical tumours.

Germline mutations of the adenomatosis polyposis coli (APC) tumour suppressor gene, located on chromosome 5q21, cause most cases of FAP. APC is a large, multifunctional protein which interacts with a number of other proteins including β–catenin, glycogen synthase kinase-3β (GSK3β), axin, E-cadherin and tubulin. The key interaction is with β–catenin, an important transcription factor in the WNT signalling pathway, as APC regulates the degradation of β–catenin and thereby downstream WNT signalling. Wild-type APC forms a cytoplasmic complex with β–catenin and GSK3β that leads to β–catenin degradation whereas mutant APC results in reduced β–catenin degradation and a subsequent increase in free β–catenin, which can enter the nucleus and act as a transcription factor (Figure 1.1).

More than 70% of patients with classical FAP phenotype have identifiable germline APC mutations with many of the remaining cases due to new mutations. Germline mutations are spread throughout the gene with mutation hot spots at codons 1061 and 1309 accounting for over one-third of cases. Over 95% are nonsense or frameshift mutations resulting in premature truncation of the protein product and altered function. There is some association between the genotype i.e. the position of the mutation, and the clinical phenotype observed. However, patients with the same mutation may display different phenotypes and therefore the genotype-phenotype association is not complete.

1.6 Attenuated FAP (AFAP) and MYH associated polyposis (MAP)

Attenuated FAP refers to a clinical phenotype with less than 100 adenomas and features such as rectal sparing, later development of adenomas and carcinomas, and fewer extracolonic features than are noted in classical FAP. AFAP accounts for approximately 8% of polyposis cases and diagnostic criteria have recently been proposed. APC mutations have been noted in approximately 25% of AFAP cases and mainly occur in exon 9 or at the 5' or 3' ends of the APC gene. However, the distribution of mutations does not entirely explain the milder disease phenotype.

Germline mutations in the oxidative repair gene MYH (MutY homologue) result in a recessively inherited syndrome of multiple adenomas and an increased risk of CRC. Patients with MYH germline mutations develop sporadic mutations in APC consisting of transversions of guanine-cytosine pairs for thymine-adenine base pairs. A number of germline MYH mutations have been noted but there are two common variants—Y165C and G382D. Biallelic MYH mutations have been estimated to account for ~0.5% of incident colorectal cancer cases; cause 7.5–13.2% of classical FAP, and ~30% of AFAP cases. Screening colonoscopy has been recommended every 2 years starting at age 18–20 for both AFAP and MAP.

Figure 1.1 APC, β-catenin and WNT signalling

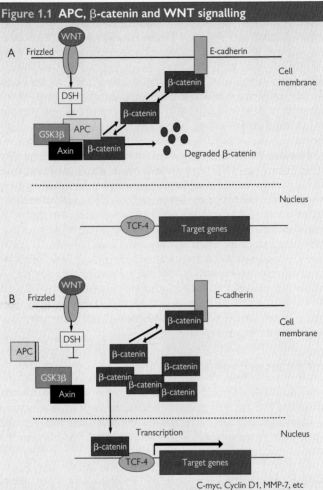

A – Normal cells: GSK3β, axin and APC form a complex promoting the degradation of free cytosolic β-catenin. WNT signalling through the frizzled receptor and dishevelled (DSH) protein inhibit APC mediated degradation of β-catenin. Much of the cellular β-catenin is bound to E-cadherin and little enters the nucleus to act as a transcription factor.

B – Tumour cells: APC mutation results in reduced degradation and increased free-cytosolic β-catenin. β-catenin relocates to the nucleus where binding to TCF-4 promoter sites results in transcriptional activation of target genes such as c-myc.

1.6.1 Lynch syndrome (LS)

Lynch syndrome is an autosomal dominant condition characterized by microsatellite instability (MSI) and an increased risk of colorectal, endometrial, and a range of other cancers (e.g. urinary tract, ovary, gastric, breast, small bowel, pancreatic-biliary, and brain tumours). LS was formerly known as Hereditary Non-Polyposis Colon Cancer

(HNPCC) but this terminology was felt to be a misnomer given the associations with multiple other tumour types.

Microsatellite are short DNA repeat sequences found throughout the genome which are repaired by mismatch repair (MMR) proteins. MMR deficient cells rapidly accumulate mutations in a large number of genes, particularly those containing microsatellite sequences. Up to 60% of LS cases have identifiable germline mutations in MMR genes with over 90% of mutations occurring in MLH1 and MSH2. Mutations in other MMR genes such as MSH6, and PMS2 are uncommon. Patients carrying a germline mutation have an 80% lifetime risk of developing colorectal cancer and contribute 2.2–4% of all CRC cases. Standardized MSI testing is performed on a panel of five mono- and di-nucleotide microsatellite repeats with tumours demonstrating instability in at least two of the five loci classified as MSI-High (MSI-H) and stability at all loci as Microsatellite Stable (MSS).

LS patients develop CRC at an early age (mean age ~44 years) and are at increased risk of synchronous and metachronous tumours. Tumours are more likely to be right sided (70% proximal to splenic flexure), poorly differentiated, mucinous, have diploid DNA content and a lymphocytic infiltrate. Clinical diagnosis is based on the Amsterdam criteria (Table 1.1) although less stringent (and more clinically useful) criteria have also been developed (i.e. Amsterdam II, Modified Amsterdam and Bethesda).

Screening colonoscopies to identify adenomas and carcinomas are advocated at 2 yearly intervals from age 25, or 5 years less than the age of onset of the first case, whichever comes first, and reduces CRC development and related deaths. In CRC cases a subtotal colectomy is normally performed due to the risk of metachronous cancers with continued surveillance of the rectal remnant required. Screening for stomach or endometrial cancers should also occur if they have occurred within a family.

1.7 Hamartomatous polyposis syndromes

Juvenile Polyposis (JP) and Peutz-Jeghers syndrome (PJS) are two rare, autosomal dominant conditions defined by the presence of hamartomatous polyps. JP affects at most 1 in 100,000 individuals and causes ~0.1% of CRC. Mutation or deletion of the SMAD4 and BMPR1A genes, involved in the TGF-ß pathway, have been noted in approximately 50% of JP cases. The lifetime risk of CRC is 40–60% and a risk of gastric cancer has also been noted. PJS incidence is estimated as 1 in 50,000–200,000 live births, and is defined by the presence of hamartomatous polyps and mucocutaneous pigmentation. A variety of cancers are noted and lifetime cancer risk may be as high as 85–93%. Lifetime CRC risk is ~40%, with an additional significant risk of pancreatic, stomach and breast cancers. Mutations in the

Table 1.1 Amsterdam 2 criteria and Bethesda guidelines for Lynch syndrome

Amsterdam criteria 2	Revised Bethesda guidelines
At least three relatives with CRC or a Lynch syndrome associated cancer (endometrium, small bowel, ureter or renal pelvis)	CRC diagnosed in a patient aged <50 years
One case should be a first-degree relative	Presence of synchronous, metachronous CRC or other Lynch syndrome-related tumours, regardless of age
At least two successive generations should be affected	CRC with MSI-H phenotype diagnosed in a patient aged <60 years
At least one tumour should be diagnosed before the age of 50 years	Patient with CRC and a first-degree relative with a Lynch syndrome-related tumour, with one of the cancers diagnosed at age <50 years
FAP should be excluded in the CRC case if any	Patient with CRC with two or more first-degree or second-degree relatives with a Lynch syndrome related tumour regardless of age
Tumours should be verified by histopathological examination	Lynch syndrome related tumours include colorectal, endometrial, stomach, ovarian, pancreas, ureter, renal pelvis, biliary tract, brain tumours, sebaceous gland adenomas and keratoacanthomas, and carcinoma of the small bowel.

Data from Umar 2004 and Vasen 1991.

STK11 (LKB1) gene are noted in ~60% of patients and large genomic deletions in a further ~20%. CRC surveillance, as well as for other related cancers, is recommended in both conditions.

1.8 Other genetic factors

Genome Wide Association (GWA) case control studies of familial or early onset colorectal cancer have recently provided insights into multiple low penetrance genetic loci which may contribute to the incidence of CRC. Other studies have examined the effect of polymorphisms in specific genes involved in DNA repair and cellular metabolism.

1.9 Biology of colorectal cancer

Colorectal cancers develop from early to late adenomas and then into an invasive adenocarcinoma. These pathological changes are associated with the accumulation of multiple genetic abnormalities including the inactivation of tumour suppressor genes, the activation of oncogenes, as well as multiple mutations in other genes.

1.10 Microsatellite instability (MSI) and Chromosomal Instability (CIN)

In addition to patients with Lynch syndrome approximately 15% of sporadic CRC's demonstrate MSI. Hypermethylation and silencing of the MLH1 promoter region is the most common cause in sporadic CRC, with MMR gene mutations noted less frequently. Similar to LS sporadic MMR deficient tumours tend to be right-sided, mucinous tumours with a lymphocytic infiltrate. Patients with MMR deficient cancers have a significantly improved prognosis compared to patients with MMR proficient tumours. These tumours also maintain a normal diploid DNA content but develop mutations in multiple genes including tumour suppressor genes such as TGFβ receptor II. The remaining 85% of sporadic CRC have chromosomal instability (CIN) and an aneuploid DNA content, i.e. have an abnormal chromosome number and structure with the loss of genetic material including wild-type copies of tumour suppressor genes. The development of CIN is poorly understood but mutated APC/activated WNT signalling may be important determinants.

1.11 Inactivation of tumour suppressor genes

WNT signalling is crucial in the development of CRC with APC mutations causing FAP. Mutation of APC occurs early in the development of most sporadic colorectal adenomas and cancers. Over 80% of sporadic cancers have one APC mutation and more than 60% of sporadic mutations occur in a region designated the MCR (Mutations Cluster Region) between codons 1286 and 1513 (<10% of coding region), with hotspots at codons 1309 and 1450. p53, known as the 'guardian of the genome', is a key tumour suppressor gene that, in response to cellular stress, can induce cell cycle arrest, activation of DNA repair proteins or apoptosis if DNA damage cannot be repaired. Loss of p53 function is noted in approximately 85% of CRC usually due to mutation of one allele and genomic loss of the other on chromosome 17p. Loss of p53 is typically noted at the adenoma to carcinoma transition.

Loss of chromosome 18q is seen in up to 70% of CRCs. The incidence of 18q loss progressively increases during the development of adenoma to carcinoma sequence. Common regions of genomic loss have been localized including coding regions for tumour suppressor genes DCC and Smad4.

1.12 **Activation of oncogenes**

KRAS is a GTP-binding protein with intrinsic GTPase activity located on the cytoplasmic surface of the cell membrane, which activates the PI3 Kinase and RAF-MEK-ERK pathways, with subsequent promotion of cell survival and proliferation. KRAS mutations, resulting in a constitutively activated GTPase, are seen in 40–50% of colorectal adenomas and carcinomas. Mutations in other members of these pathways including BRAF and PI3 kinase, have also been noted.

1.13 **Staging of colorectal cancer**

The Dukes' and TNM systems are the most commonly used staging tools in CRC. Cuthbert Dukes' published a staging system for rectal cancer in 1932, based on cases managed at St. Mark's Hospital, London. This classified tumours by pathological local tumour invasion into three groups (A = confined to the rectal wall; B = breached extra-rectal tissues; C = the presence of lymph node metastases) and established that the system accurately predicted prognosis. The system was subsequently modified to subdivide Dukes' stage C (C1 – localized LN metastases only; C2 – metastatic deposits up to the highest LN), adding stage D (the presence of distant metastases), and to extend the system to cover colon cancers. Dukes' staging is still frequently used given its simplicity and reproducibility.

The TNM (Tumour-Node-Stage) staging system is commonly used in clinical practice and definitions for the 'T', 'N' and "M" categories based on the 6th edition are listed in Table 1.2. The presence or absence of distant metastases can be derived from clinical, surgical or radiology assessments. Prognostic stage groups are derived from assessment of T, N, and M parameters (Table 1.3). Prescripts indicating the derivation of the data - 'c' indicating clinical/radiological classification, 'p' indicating pathological classification e.g. pT1, have been incorporated into TNM staging. A combination of clinical and pathologically derived data is usually used to derive the final stage grouping (e.g. pT3, pN0, cM0). The TNM system is regularly updated with the aim of improving staging categorization and survival estimates but changes particularly between the 5th and 6th editions has provoked criticism. This centred on changes to the classification of peri-tumoural nodules. TNM5 used a 3mm size criteria (>3mm = nodal metastasis; <3mm = vascular invasion or discontinuous tumour contributing to T stage) whereas in TNM 6 classified based on their contour ('rounded contour' = nodal metastasis; 'irregular margin' = contributing to T stage). This introduces a subjective assessment into staging with the risk of reduced reproducibility and also changes the N stage definition on which decisions regarding adjuvant chemotherapy are often based.

Table 1.2 TNM6 definitions

	Category	Definition
Primary tumour (T)	TX	Primary tumour cannot be assessed
	T0	No evidence of primary tumour
	Tis	Carcinoma in-situ (intraepithelial or intramucosal carcinoma)
	T1	Tumour invades the submucosa
	T2	Tumour invades the muscularis propria
	T3	Tumour invades through the muscularis propria into the submucosa or into the nonperitonealized pericolic or perirectal tissues
	T4	Tumour directly invades other organs or structures (T4a) or perforates the visceral peritoneum (T4b)
Regional lymph nodes (N)	NX	Regional lymph nodes cannot be assessed
	N0	No regional LN metastases
	N1	Metastases in one to three lymph nodes
	N2	Metastases in four or more lymph nodes
Distant metastases (M)	MX	Presence of distant metastases cannot be assessed
	M0	No distant metastases
	M1	Distant metastases to any non-regional lymph node, any distant organ or tissue, and/or peritoneum, positive cytology from peritoneal or pleural cavity

Based on TNM atlas, Wiley 2005.

The Royal College of Pathologists (UK) have recommended the continued use of TNM5 given these and other concerns regarding the changes introduced in TNM6. The seventh edition of TNM staging has recently been introduced and the changes in this compared with TNM6 are outlined in Table 1.4. Further changes in the classification of peri-tumoural nodules have been made with the incorporation of an 'N1c' category for non-nodal satellite deposits. Despite this TNM5 is likely to remain the standard advocated for use in the UK.

TNM staging does not include an assessment of the effects of treatment strategy on outcomes. The prescript 'y' e.g. ypT ypN, has

Table 1.3 TNM stage groups and survival rates using 5th and 6th editions

			AJCC TNM 5th Edition		AJCC TNM 6th Edition	
			Stage	5-year Survival	Stage	5-year Survival
T1/T2	N0	M0	Stage 1	93.2%	Stage 1	93.2%
T3	N0	M0	Stage 2	82.5%	Stage 2a	84.7%
T4	N0	M0			Stage 2b	72.2%
T1/T2	N1	M0	Stage 3	59.5%	Stage 3a	83.4%
T3/T4	N1	M0			Stage 3b	64.1%
Any T	N2	M0			Stage 3c	44.3%
Any T	Any N	M1	Stage 4	8.1%	Stage 4	8.1%

Data from O'Connell 2004.

Table 1.4 Changes to TNM between versions 6 and 7

		Version 6		Version 7	
Primary tumour	T1	Tumour invades the subserosa		Tumour invades the subserosa	
	T2	Tumour invades the muscularis propria		Tumour invades the muscularis propria	
	T3	Tumour invades through the muscularis propria into the submucosa or into the nonperitonealized pericolic or perirectal tissues		Tumour invades through the muscularis propria into the submucosa or into the nonperitonealized pericolic or perirectal tissues	
	T4	T4a	directly invades other organs or structures	T4a	tumour perforates the visceral peritoneum or
		T4b	tumour perforates the visceral peritoneum	T4b	directly invades other organs or structures

(Continued)

Table 1.4 (Contd.)

		Version 6	Version 7	
Regional lymph nodes	N0	No regional LN metastases	No regional LN metastases	
	N1	Metastasis in 1 to 3 nodes	N1a	1 node
			N1b	2–3 nodes
			N1c	satellites in subserosa without regional nodes
	N2	Metastasis in 4 or more nodes	N2a	4–6 nodes
			N2b	7 or more nodes
Distant metastases	M0	No distant metastases	No distant metastases	
	M1	Distant metastases	M1a	one organ
			M1b	more than one organ or peritoneum

Based on TNM atlas, Wiley 2005.

been incorporated to indicate that neo-adjuvant (pre-operative) treatment has been given and may have altered a tumours pathological appearance and staging. This is mainly used in patients with rectal cancer where pre-operative short course radiotherapy or long course chemoradiotherapy are standard treatments. The plane of surgical excision of rectal cancer and presence of tumour at the circumferential resection margin (CRM) has been significantly associated with the risk of local recurrence in rectal cancer, and routine assessment of the CRM although not part of TNM staging system is recommended.

Suggested reading

Chow E, Thirlwell C, Macrae F, and Lipton L (2004) Colorectal cancer and inherited mutations in base-excision repair. *Lancet Oncol*, **5**: 600–6.

De Vita VT, Hellman S and Rosenberg SA (2001). *Cancer: Principles and Practice of Oncology*. Sixth Edition. Sections 7 & 8—Cancers of the Colon and Rectum. pp 1216–1319.

Fearnhead NS, Britton MP, and Bodmer WF (2001) The ABC of APC. *Hum Mol Gen*, **10**(7): 721–33.

Knudsen AL, Bisgaard ML, and Bulow S (2003) Attenuated familial adenomatous polyposis (AFAP). A review of the literature. *Fam Cancer*, **2**: 43–55.

Norat T, Bingham S, Ferrari P, et al. (2005) Meat, Fish, and Colorectal Cancer Risk: The European Prospective Investigation into Cancer and Nutrition. *J Natl Cancer Inst*, **97**: 906–16.

O'Connell JB, Maggard MA, Ko CY (2004) Colon Cancer Survival Rates With the New American Joint Committee on Cancer Sixth Edition Staging. *Journal of the National Cancer Institute*, **96**(19): 1420–5.

Umar A, Boland CR, Terdiman JP, et al. (2004) Revised Bethesda Guidelines for hereditary nonpolyposis colorectal cancer (Lynch syndrome) and microsatellite instability. *J Natl Cancer Inst*, **96**(4): 261–8.

Vasen HF, Mecklin JP, Khan PM, Lynch HT (1991) The International Collaborative Group on Hereditary Non-Polyposis Colorectal Cancer (ICG-HNPCC). *Diseases of the Colon and Rectum*, **34**(5): 424–5.

Chapter 2

Screening and diagnosis of colorectal cancer

Kai J. Leong and Dion Morton

Key points

- Screening is effective in reducing colorectal cancer deaths in an average risk population
- Screening strategy for increased risk individuals involves risk stratification on the basis of family history, the detection of genetic mutations, or the duration of disease for patients with pancolitis
- Newer screening options appear promising and have the potential to either replace or act as adjuncts to current screening modalities
- Less than a third of patients with colorectal cancers present with symptoms that are independently associated with the disease
- Colonoscopy is the gold standard investigation for suspected colorectal cancer but is associated with some significant risks.

Colorectal cancer (CRC) fulfils the criteria set out by the World Health Organization as a condition worthy of screening. The prospect of reducing mortality and increasing detection of early disease has prompted the introduction of national screening programmes for CRC in many countries.

This chapter aims to provide an evidence-based summary of screening strategies and options for those with average and increased risk of developing CRC and to highlight some of the diagnostic strategies being practised in the UK.

2.1 Screening for at risk population

2.1.1 Inherited colorectal cancer

2.1.1.1 High penetrance autosomal dominant disease

Individuals with family history that fulfils empiric criteria, presence of pathognomonic clinical features, and/or identification of known genetic defect in affected relatives have a 30–50% life time risk of developing CRC. They should be referred to Regional Genetics Centres for counselling and consideration for gene specific, direct mutation analysis.

2.1.1.2 Familial Adenomatous Polyposis (FAP)

Testing

Genetic screening for FAP typically begins with a Protein Truncating Test (PTT). Mutations are detected in about 80% of families and facilitate predictive testing for at risk family members. Colonoscopy surveillance is provided from the early teens for all at risk and affected family members, enabling planned prophylactic surgery, usually by the age of 20 years. A new autosomal recessive condition, MYH is associated with multiple large bowel adenomas (usually more than 20) and so mimics attenuated FAP (see Chapter 1).

Surveillance

Following surgery, life-long annual sigmoidoscopy surveillance on the anorectal cuff (panproctocolectomy) or retained rectum (subtotal colectomy) will be required. FAP is also associated with the development of periampullary adenomas and progression to periampullary carcinoma. Consequently 3 yearly Upper GI Endoscopy, using a side viewing endoscope to inspect the second part of the duodenum, is recommended for individuals over the age of 30. Unlike large bowel surveillance, evidence demonstrating benefit from regular upper GI surveillance is lacking. However, duodenal cancer is an increasing risk to FAP families, as prophylactic surgery for colorectal cancer becomes more effectively implemented.

Hereditary Non-polyposis Colorectal Cancer (HNPCC)/Lynch Syndrome
Testing

This autosomal dominant syndrome is caused by germline mutation in genes encoding the mismatch repair (MMR) system (MLH1, MSH2, PMS2 and MSH6), leading to loss of mismatch repair proteins in the tumour and associated failure of DNA repair. This enables testing of tumour samples either by immunohistochemistry (IHC) or by microsatellite instability (MSI) test.

Following a positive test, the affected individual is invited to undergo germline mutation testing. Once identified, direct mutation testing can then be performed for at risk family members. The clinical criteria for MMR gene testing have been broadened to increase the identification of families affected (Revised Bethesda guidelines, see Chapter 1, Table 1.1).

Up to 20% of sporadic CRC can have deficiency in MMR proteins, but this is most commonly due to promoter methylation of MLH1. This somatic inactivation of MMR genes in CRCs means that less than 20% will be associated HNPCC. Tumour testing is therefore restricted by clinical (Bethesda) criteria to minimize testing of non-HNPCC patients.

Surveillance

Biennial colonoscopic surveillance at the age of 25 or 5 years younger than the age of the first case in the family, whichever is earlier is recommended. Surveillance should continue up to the age of 75 or when they are proven non gene-carrier.

Total colectomy with ileorectal anastomosis should be offered to those with evidence of progressive colonic neoplasia, reducing the risk of metachronous cancers. Life-long sigmodoscopic surveillance of the rectum will be required. Because of the significant increased risk of endometrial and ovarian cancers in HNPCC families, surveillance by annual ultrasound, smear test, and tumour markers is offered, and prophylactic hysterectomy considered upon completion of family.

Peutz-Jeghers Syndrome (PJS)

Individuals with this rare autosomal dominant condition are at risk of developing cancers at multiple sites; the most prevalent being within the small bowel, colorectum, pancreas, breast, ovarian, cervical, and prostate. Small bowel surveillance can be achieved with MR/CT enterocolysis or capsule endoscopy. Colorectal cancer surveillance with colonoscopy is recommended 3 yearly in adults. Data on the benefit of screening in other organs is limited.

Juvenile Polyposis Syndrome (JPS)

Individuals with JPS are at an increased risk of developing colorectal cancer. Large bowel surveillance is provided on an empirical basis by colonoscopy from the late teens. As with PJS, surveillance is greatly complicated by the presence of multiple non-neoplastic polyps.

2.1.2 Familial clustering

Individuals in this group have a family history of CRC, usually with an autosomal dominant pattern of inheritance, accounting for up to 30% of CRC risk. Risk of CRC, in the absence of genetic testing, is assessed using data from large population-based studies and increases with greater number of family members affected, and the age at diagnosis. Colonoscopy is the screening modality of choice for this group. Based upon empirical risk tables, surveillance is offered from five yearly to one-off colonoscopy. Low penetrance CRC susceptibility alleles have been identified and CRC risk for individuals who have inherited these alleles are now quantifiable. This could enable better risk stratification and the potential to exclude low risk family members. Such testing could be incorporated into population based screening programmes.

2.2 Screening for average risk population

2.2.1 Faecal Occult Blood Testing (FOBT)

There are two types of FOBT in common use:

- Guaiac-based test (G-FOBT)—detects the pseudoperoxidise activity of haemoglobin in faeces and is not specific for human blood
- Immunochemical-based tests (I-FOBT)—utilizes one or more antibodies that are specific to human haemoglobin.

G-FOBT has been shown to reduce colorectal cancer mortality in 4 large population-based randomized controlled trials (RCT) after more than 10 years of follow up (Table 2.1). The results from the UK and Denmark were directly comparable. The apparent improved results in the US trial were ascribed to a far higher colonoscopy rate, which in turn was due to more frequent FOB testing and a lower positive test threshold.

G-FOBT has a relatively low sensitivity (10.8–16.7%) in detecting colorectal neoplasia and can be affected by certain food. I-FOBTs have been developed to increase the sensitivity and to eliminate the influence of dietary factors. Studies have reported improved sensitivity of I-FOBT over G-FOBT but results from large comparative population based studies are awaited.

Table 2.1 Characteristics, Relative Risk (RR) and Confidence Interval (CI) of 4 RCT using FOBT

Study	Country	Screening frequency	Age Range (yr)	Follow up period (yr)	RR	95% CI
Funen	Denmark	Annual	45–75	17	0.84	0.73–0.96
		Biennial			0.89	0.78–1.01
Minnesota	U.S.	Annual	50–80	18	0.67	0.51–0.83
		Biennial			0.79	0.62–0.97
Nottingham	U.K.	Biennial	45–74	11.7	0.87	0.78–0.97
Goteberg	Sweden	Biennial	60–64	19	0.84	0.71–0.99

Data from Hewitson et al. (2008) Am J Gastroenterol **103**: 1541–9.

The NHS Bowel Cancer Screening Programme offers G-FOBT every 2 years to anyone aged between 60–69 years old. Individuals with positive results will be invited for colonoscopies. In the US, G-FOBT and I-FOBT are two of the screening tools recommended. Individuals from the age of 50 are invited for annual screening using FOBTs.

2.2.2 Flexible sigmoidoscopy

Flexible sigmoidoscopy enables the distal colon and rectum to be visualized and adenomas to be removed, preventing malignancy developing. The efficacy of this examination is enhanced because two thirds of sporadic colorectal cancers develop within reach of the sigmoidoscope. The ability to identify individuals who harbour proximal lesions not reached by flexible sigmoidoscopy would enhance its efficacy. Features of distal adenomas that are associated with proximal lesions are:

- Villous morphology
- High grade dysplasia
- ≥ 1 cm in diameter
- ≥ 3 adenomas.

Individuals with these features would require colonoscopy.

A recent RCT in the UK demonstrated that screening with 'once only' flexible sigmoidoscopy resulted in reduction in CRC incidence and mortality by 23% and 31% respectively after a median follow-up of 11 years.

2.2.3 Colonoscopy

Colonoscopy is regarded as the gold standard investigation for the detection of colorectal polyps and cancer. Currently, it is the final investigation following all positive screening tests. Screening with colonoscopy is safe and feasible. Case-control studies have demonstrated reduction in CRC incidence and mortality but it has not been evaluated in population-based RCT.

Colonoscopy as a primary screening tool is recommended in the US and in Germany but the cost effectiveness of colonoscopy has not been demonstrated. The resource implications are considerable and it would be undeliverable through existing endoscopy facilities in the UK.

2.2.4 Novel diagnostic options

2.2.4.1 CT colonography (CTC)/Virtual colonoscopy

This advance imaging technique combines the use of helical computer tomography and complex rendering programmes to generate 2-dimensional and 3-dimensional images of the colon and rectum.

Full bowel preparation is required. Images are taken in the prone and supine positions after rectal insufflation. Its main advantage is its non-invasiveness. Evidence of its role as a screening tool is limited.

Most studies evaluated its performance in selected mixed symptomatic and presymptomatic patients. CTC has reported sensitivity of ≥90% and specificity of >85% for detecting ≥ 1 cm neoplastic lesions in average risk asymptomatic patients. To date, there is only one RCT and its report is awaited (SIGGAR 1). This trial, however, examines the diagnostic performance of CTC against barium enema and colonoscopy in symptomatic patients.

2.2.4.2 Stool-extracted DNA assays

This non-invasive screening test has been designed to improve the performance of FOBTs. It works on the premise that epithelial cells of adenomas and cancers are continually shed into stool which allows detection of a series of gene mutations in stool-extracted DNA. One large cohort study which compared the performance of stool DNA testing and FOBT in CRC screening, found stool DNA testing had greater sensitivity of detecting high risk polyps (18.2% vs. 10.8%) and cancers (51.6% vs. 12.9%) without compromising specificity (94.4% vs. 95.2%). This promising test would need to be evaluated in population-based diagnostic trial before being taken forward as a screening tool.

2.2.4.3 Proteomics

Proteomics use mass spectrometry-based protein analysis technologies such as MALDI-TOF and SELDI-TOF to distinguish protein patterns and profiles of individuals with cancer and those without. It is generally non-invasive; analysing proteins from easily accessible body fluids such as urine and blood. Early studies in CRC have been promising; reporting sensitivities of 65–89% and specificities of 83–90%. Like many novel techniques, data on its reproducibility is lacking. Independent validation studies are still required.

2.3 Clinical Presentations of CRC

Before the screening era, most of CRC diagnoses made in asymptomatic individuals were incidental. Often, by the time patients become symptomatic, their cancers have become advanced. Less than 9% of all CRC in England between 1996–2002 were Duke's A. In contrast, UK pilot screening studies reported that 49–62% of screen-detected tumours were Duke's A.

Symptoms that are independently associated with CRC are:

- Rectal bleeding
- Change in bowel habit
- Weight loss
- Abdominal pain
- Diarrhoea
- Constipation
- Microcytic anaemia.

However, less than a third of CRC patients have these symptoms. About 15% of CRC patients will present as surgical emergency with acute bowel obstruction and/or perforation. Their 5 year survival is substantially worse than their counterparts who present electively.

2.4 Investigations

2.4.1 Lower GI endoscopy
Flexible sigmoidoscopy can identify up to two thirds of all colorectal cancers. It may be suitable for patients presenting with fresh rectal bleeding. If cancer is found, full visualization of the colon is needed to identify synchronous lesions. In most UK hospitals, the investigation of choice for full colonic visualization is colonoscopy. It has the added advantage of being able to 'tattoo' tumours to aid identification during laparoscopic surgery. However, the completion rates vary among centres and its complications, though low, is not insignificant. The overall risk of perforation is in the order of 0.082% and this risk doubles if polypectomy is performed.

2.4.2 Radiological imaging
Alternatives to colonoscopy include double contrast barium enema and CT colonography (CTC). A large prospective study on symptomatic patients found that barium enema has comparable sensitivity (48% vs. 59%) and specificity (90% vs. 96%) as CTC for the detection of lesions >1 cm but both modalities were inferior to colonoscopy (sensitivity 98%, specificity >99%). When smaller lesions were considered, the performance of barium enema and CTC decreased even further. Results of the SIGGAR 1 trial comparing CTC and barium enema in symptomatic patients, due this year, will provide further insight into the performance characteristics of these two modalities.

2.5 'Straight to test' clinics

These were introduced in 2005 with the aim of improving cancer waiting times in the NHS and consequently, utilizing urgent and routine clinic appointments more efficiently. Patients referred to a specialist with symptoms of suspected cancer would undergo diagnostic investigations in the first instance before being seen in hospital. Data from the Leicester Colorectal Group has demonstrated improvement in waiting times following the introduction of the STT clinic, but no patient outcome data has been reported. Suggested investigations according to presenting symptoms are shown in Table 2.2.

Table 2.2 Suggested diagnostic investigations according to presenting symptoms			
Presenting symptoms	Age	Diagnostic investigations	
		1st line	Alternative
Rectal bleeding and change in bowel habit ≥6 weeks	≥40 years	Colonoscopy	Flexible sigmoidoscopy and barium enema, CTC
Rectal bleeding without anal symptoms	Recommended over 60 years; Discretionary over 45 years	Flexible sigmodoscopy	
Change in bowel habit	Over 60 years	Colonoscopy	Barium enma, CTC
Palpable abdominal mass	All ages	CT abdomen	Ultrasound scan
Palpable rectal mass	All ages	Sigmoidoscopy (Rigid/Flexible) and biopsy	
Unexplained iron deficiency anaemia Men ≤11g/100 ml Non-menstruating women ≤10g/100ml	All ages	Barium enem + OGD	Colonoscopy, CTC

Data from Hemingway, Jameson, and Kelly (2006) *Colorectal Disease* **8**: 289–95.

Suggested reading

Atkin, W.S., Edwards, R., Kralj-Hans, I. et al. (2010) Once-only flexible sigmoidoscopy screening in prevention of colorectal cancer: a multicentre randomised controlled trial. *Lancet* **375**(9726): 1624–33.

Dunlop, M.G. (2002) Guidance on gastrointestinal surveillance for hereditary non-polyposis colorectal cancer, familial adenomatous polypolis, juvenile polyposis, and Peutz-Jeghers syndrome. *Gut* **51**(5): V21–7.

Hemingway, D.M., Jameson, J. & Kelly, M. J. (2006) Straight to test: introduction of a city-wide protocol driven investigation of suspected colorectal cancer. *Colorectal Dis* **8**: 289–95.

The Association of Coloproctology of Great Britain and Ireland (2007). Guidelines for the Management of Colorectal Cancer, 3rd Edition. Available at: http://www.acpgbi.org.uk/assets/documents/ COLO_guides.pdf. Accessed on 31 May 2010.

UK Flexible Sigmoidoscopy Screening Trial Investigators (2002) Single flexible sigmoidoscopy screening to prevent colorectal cancer: baseline findings of a UK multicentre randomised trial. *Lancet* **359**: 1291–1300.

UK Colorectal Cancer Screening Pilot Group (2004) Results of the first round of a demonstration pilot of screening for colorectal cancer in the United Kingdom. *BMJ* **329**: 133.

Umar, A., Boland, C.R., Terdiman, J.P. et al. (2004) Revised Bethesda Guidelines for hereditary nonpolyposis colorectal cancer (Lynch syndrome) and microsatellite instability. *J Natl Cancer Inst* **96**: 261–8.

Chapter 3

Surgical management of colorectal cancer

Zahirul Huq and Dominic Slade

Key points

- Oncological principles for colorectal cancer surgery involve removal of the tumour with an adequate margin and clearance of the draining lymphatic basin
- Laparoscopic colorectal surgery offers several advantages over the equivalent open procedure. Laparoscopic resection should be considered as an alternative to open resection for individuals in whom both techniques are suitable
- The gold standard of rectal cancer surgery is dissection in the TME plane
- Early (T1) rectal cancers may be adequately treated by TEMS
- A 'cylindrical' abdominoperineal resection is oncologically superior to the conventional technique for low T3 and T4 rectal cancers especially with the pelvic floor involvement.

3.1 Principles

Surgery for colorectal cancer is founded upon two key principles, resection of the tumour with an adequate margin and clearance of its entire lymphatic drainage based on its arterial blood supply. The extent of resection is therefore determined by the number of arteries requiring division in order to adequately remove all the lymphatics of the tumour-bearing colon.

3.2 Colon cancer operative management

For cancers affecting the caecum, ascending colon, hepatic flexure and proximal transverse colon a right hemicolectomy is usually performed. This involves ligation of the ileocolic, right colic and right branch of the middle colic arteries as close to their origins as possible. With left-sided cancers affecting the descending and sigmoid colon some surgeons prefer to divide the inferior mesenteric artery at its origin and anastomose the colon on to the top of the rectum. The resulting anastomosis relies heavily on blood supply from the colonic marginal artery that can at times be tenuous. Consequently some surgeons prefer to preserve the inferior mesenteric artery taking the left branch of the middle colic, ascending and desecending left colic arteries and creating an anastomosis to the sigmoid colon. Transverse colon cancers situated in the distal two thirds, including the splenic flexure, may also be managed by extended right or left hemicolectomy, the former involving division of the middle colic artery at its origin in addition to the arterial divisions required for a right hemicolectomy. The choice is influenced by tumour site, surgical preference, and presumed functional outcome.

3.3 Colon cancer-radical surgery

Recently a group of surgeons from Erlangen, Germany have shown that more radical dissection to include the entire mesocolic package based on embryological planes equivalent to the principle of mesorectal dissection in rectal cancer surgery, improves 5 year colonic cancer survival rates by as much as 6.5% without a significant increase in perioperative mortality or morbidity. The completeness of the mesocolic resection will be prospectively evaluated in the FOXTROT trial, a multicentre randomized phase III trial of neoadjuvant versus adjuvant chemotherapy in colon cancer.

3.3.1 En bloc resection

If an adjacent organ is involved with a colonic tumour then it is important that part or all of that organ is removed en bloc with the colonic tumour to prevent tumour disruption and cell spillage. Tumours involving the sigmoid colon or rectum may result in multivisceral resections of colon with bladder and prostate in men, or uterus in women. Careful preoperative staging and planning with a multidisciplinary team is essential to ensure a curative resection.

3.3.2 Laparoscopic colorectal surgery

Laparoscopic colorectal surgery offers both short and long-term advantages over the equivalent open operation and where appropriate is becoming the standard operative approach.

3.3.3 Advantages of laparoscopic surgery

Early benefits relate to better pulmonary function, less pain, reduced analgesic requirement and faster recovery in the post-operative period. The adequacy of oncological resection and lymph node harvest is equivalent to open surgery as demonstrated by both the CLASICC trial and a more recent high quality multi-centre German trial (LAPKON II). There is also less intra-operative blood loss, quicker return of gut function, superior cosmesis and a reduction in wound infection rates (of up to 50%). Long-term benefits relate to a lower incidence of adhesive intestinal obstruction.

3.3.4 Potential drawbacks of laparoscopic surgery

Laparoscopic colorectal surgery has a very steep learning curve and mastery can take many years. Notably the CLASICC trial demonstrated a difference in the circumferential margin positivity rate for rectal tumours, with twice as many patients in the laparoscopic group (12%) having an involved circumferential margin compared to the open surgery group (6%). This difference was not statistically significant, and follow up in the short term has not shown an increased rate of local recurrence in the laparoscopic surgery group. Despite the favourable outcomes of a laparoscopic resection it can not be considered a panacea for all colorectal tumours. The bulky low rectal tumour lying within a narrow pelvis continues to provide a stern challenge to the most able surgeon, due to ease of access, specimen retraction and limitations in the laparoscopic tools (e.g. laparoscopic cross-stapling devices). Some studies have reported anastomotic leak rates approaching 20% following laparoscopic anterior resection.

3.4 Rectal cancer

The management of rectal tumours has continued to evolve over the last two decades due to technical advances in anastomotic stapling devices and improvements in our understanding of mesorectal lymphatic and embryological anatomy, tumour biology, and developments in adjuvant and neoadjuvant therapies. A tumour is classified as rectal if its distal margin is 15cms or less from the anal verge on rigid sigmoidoscopy. Rectal tumours can be further classified as upper, mid and lower in terms of position based on distances of 11–15 cm, 6–10 cm and <6 cm from the anal verge respectively. Upper and mid rectal cancers are usually treated by anterior resection alone. In comparison low rectal tumours may be surgically managed by carrying out a low anterior resection or an abdomino-perineal resection (APR). The choice of operation depends upon tumour characteristics and patient factors.

3.4.1 **Total mesorectal excision (TME)**

Operative technique is of paramount importance in the management of rectal cancers and has measurable prognostic implications in terms of local recurrence. Precise dissection under direct vision within a loose, largely avascular, areolar plane lying between the visceral fascia or mesorectum and parietal fascia, commonly referred to as the TME (total mesorectal excision) plane, has been popularized by Heald (Figure 3.1). Rates of local tumour recurrence with TME have been reported to be as low as 4% after 5 years in comparison to rates as high as 45% where mesorectal disruption has occurred.

Quirke analysed multiple TME specimens and observed that mesorectal tumour spread is less than 5 cm distal to the tumour margin. Accordingly for upper rectal cancers it can be argued that a total mesorectal excision is unnecessary, allowing the rectum to be transected at a higher level without compromising oncological out-comes. This approach has considerable advantages in terms of better post-operative bowel function, and reduced anastomotic leak rates. In contrast, mid and low rectal cancers require complete mesorectal excision to maximize the chances of adequate local tumour clearance.

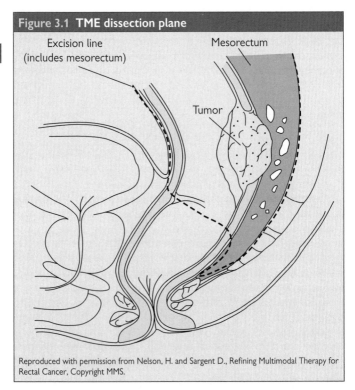

Figure 3.1 TME dissection plane

Excision line (includes mesorectum)

Mesorectum

Tumor

Reproduced with permission from Nelson, H. and Sargent D., Refining Multimodal Therapy for Rectal Cancer, Copyright MMS.

3.4.2 Rectal cancer recurrence and good surgical technique

The influence of total mesorectal excision on outcomes is neatly demonstrated by two large European neoadjuvant radiotherapy trials often quoted for their impact on rectal cancer. The Swedish Rectal Cancer Trial where surgical technique was not standardized, reported a 27% 5 year local recurrence rate for the surgery-alone arm and 11% in those who received additional preoperative short course radiotherapy. By today's standards even the latter recurrence rate would be considered too high. In contrast the 'Dutch Trial', founded on a standardized TME dissection, demonstrated a 2-year local recurrence rate of 8.2% in the surgery alone group illustrating the importance of good quality surgery on disease-free survival.

Subgroup analysis of the Dutch trial data showed tumour height and TNM stage to be significant predictors of local recurrence. The addition of neoadjuvant radiotherapy to surgery had the greatest benefit for mid rectal tumours. More recently the UK MRC CRO7 trial demonstrated a 3 year local recurrence rate of 4% with neoadjuvant radiotherapy independent of tumour height.

3.4.3 Surgical strategies for low rectal cancer

Low rectal cancers may be successfully managed by more than one operative approach and the correct one depends on the stage, position and anatomical relationship of the tumour to the pelvic floor and sphincter complex as well as the likely healing and functional outcome of a low anastomosis. The choices are:

- Low anterior resection (usually with stapled coloanal anastomosis)
- Ultra Low anterior resection (resulting from an additional intersphincteric dissection/mucosectomy and creation of a hand sewn coloanal anastomosis)
- Abdominoperineal resection (resulting in a permanent end colostomy).

The first two operations restore intestinal continuity with either a straight end-to-end or end to side coloanal anastomosis, or by fashioning a colon 'J' pouch prior to its anastomosis onto the anal canal. Another strategy is the transverse coloplasty which involves making a longitudinal colotomy approximately 8 cm in length and 3–4 cm proximal to the distal end of the colon. This colotomy is then closed transversely, and the distal end of the colon is anastomosed to the anus. A Cochrane review of reconstructive techniques after rectal cancer resection identified nine randomized controlled trials (RCTs, n = 473) that compared straight coloanal anastomosis to the colonic J pouch. Up to 18 months postoperatively, the colonic J pouch was superior to a straight coloanal anastomosis in most studies with respect to bowel frequency, urgency, faecal incontinence and use of antidiarrheal medication. There were too few patients with long-term bowel function outcomes to determine if this advantage continued after 18 months postoperatively. Four RCTs (n = 215) compared the side-to-end anastomosis to the colonic J pouch. These studies showed no difference in bowel function outcomes between these two techniques. Similarly, three RCTs (n = 158) compared transverse coloplasty to colonic J pouch. Similarly, there were no differences in bowel function outcomes in these small studies. Overall, there were no significant differences in postoperative complications with any of the anastomotic strategies.

3.4.4 **Complications**

Construction of a difficult colorectal or coloanal anastomosis is associated with significant risk of leakage. Pelvic anastomoses above the peritoneal reflection have a reported leak rate of 1.5% compared to 6.6% for those below. Leak rates from an ultra-low anterior resection are even higher (8%) and can result in the creation of a stoma that frequently becomes permanent. Fashioning a defunctioning stoma (ileostomy/colostomy) has been shown to considerably decrease the incidence of symptomatic leakage requiring surgery. Anastomotic leakage following a rectal cancer resection can adversely influence 5-year local recurrence and overall survival, with rates of 11–25% and 54% respectively. Furthermore, rectal tumour perforation (at presentation or iatrogenic) is associated with an increased rate of local recurrence (25–50% at 5 years).

3.4.5 **Hartmann's procedure**

Following resection of a sigmoid colonic or rectal tumour, a primary anastomosis may be considered unsafe. Anyone with significant cardiovascular and respiratory co-morbidities may be at increased risk of an anastomotic leak. In particular patients presenting with an obstructing distal tumour with gross proximal dilatation or perforation with contamination are at significant risk of anastomotic dehiscence. Elderly patients with compromised anal sphincter function may develop debilitating faecal incontinence following restoration of bowel continuity. Advanced rectal tumours where margin clearance has not been achieved are associated with higher rates of anastomotic failure due to local disease progression. In these situations due consideration should be given to the formation of an end colostomy and closure of the rectal stump—Hartmann's procedure. Re-anastomosis at a later date may be appropriate but in the majority of cancer cases the colostomy is permanent because of the factors that precluded a primary anastomosis in the first place.

3.4.6 **Transanal endoscopic microsurgery (TEMS)**

TEMS allows the surgeon to operate transanally using a specialized resectoscope through which instruments can be introduced akin to single incision laparoscopic surgery. Before considering whether a patient is suitable for TEMS precise preoperative assessment of stage, distance from the anal verge and circumferential position is essential. TEMS can be used as curative treatment for mobile, small T1 mid to low rectal cancers, or for patients with localized rectal cancer irrespective of metastases who are unfit for more radical open surgery. Post-operatively the treatment can be augmented by radiotherapy and chemotherapy, but long-term outcomes are unknown. A UK multicentre phase II trial of TEMS plus radiotherapy for stage I rectal cancer is currently is planned.

3.5 **Abdominoperineal resection**

3.5.1 **Background**
For rectal tumours deemed too low to perform an anastomosis or involving the pelvic floor or sphincter complex the operation of choice is an abdominoperineal resection. The inferior mesenteric artery is divided at its origin, the colon transected and the proximal sigmoid brought out as end colostomy. The rectum is dissected in the TME plane down to the pelvic floor at which point a perineal incision is made and continued until the two dissections meet allowing removal of the entire specimen through the perineum. A recent retrospective audit of a UK population-based dataset of patients with rectal cancer (1998–2004) recorded a historic abdominoperineal resection rate of 30%. By today's standards the rate is high and causative factors including low-volume surgeons (less than seven rectal resections per year), male sex, and low socioeconomic class were noted. The permanent stoma rate fell during the study period to 23% and independent experts have suggested that this is due to the emerging subspecialization of colorectal surgery (increasing the likelihood of a low anastomosis) and the influence of multidisciplinary team (MDT) discussion on management. It should however be noted that in a large proportion of patients with a low tumour there is no alternative cancer operation.

3.5.2 **The 'conventional' abdominoperineal resection**
Several studies have demonstrated a worse outcome following abdominoperineal resection than anterior resection for low rectal tumours. Local recurrence rates (36% vs. 22%); circumferential resection margin (CRM) positivity (30–41% vs. 10–12%) and 5-year cancer specific survival (38–52% vs. 57–65%) seem to favour anterior resection. Furthermore there is a higher incidence of intra-operative rectal perforation (13% vs. 2.5%) and dissection in erroneous planes following an abdominoperineal resection. Flaws in surgical technique when performing a 'conventional abdominoperineal resection' can partly explain

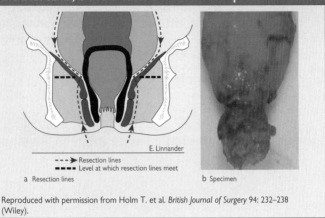

Figure 3.2 Synchronous combined abdominoperineal resection. a Dissections from above and below meet above the anal canal; b this creates a waist on the specimen

E. Linnander

- - - ▶ Resection lines
■ ■ ■ ■ Level at which resection lines meet

a Resection lines   b Specimen

Reproduced with permission from Holm T. et al. *British Journal of Surgery* 94: 232–238 (Wiley).

the differences in outcome. During this procedure the mesorectum is completely mobilized off the levator muscle thus coning in towards the top of the anal canal (Figure 3.2a). Once the perineal dissection is complete and the specimen retrieved, there inevitably is a 'waist' at the lower border of the mesorectum where the muscularis propria of the rectum is not uncommonly exposed. The 'waist' tends to coincide with the tumour location and therefore becomes a prime site where the CRM is potentially threatened (Figure 3.2b).

3.5.3 **The 'radical' abdominoperineal resection**

Holm et al. have pioneered a more radical approach with an extended perineal resection. The abdominal component of the operation remains unchanged; with one exception; the mesorectum is not dissected off the levator muscle (Figure 3.3a). However, the perineal component of the operation is carried out in the prone jack-knife position and necessitates prior abdominal closure and formation of the colostomy. Once the specimen has been retrieved, the pelvic floor defect can be closed with the aid of a myocutaneous flap, a prosthetic mesh or even primarily if the tissues can be approximated under minimal tension. The radical nature of this procedure relates to the fact that the levator muscle can be divided much further laterally, close to its origins from the pelvic side wall. In addition the coccyx is usually removed in continuity with the main specimen. The resulting specimen has a more 'cylindrical' appearance and does not possess a 'waist' due to the cuff of excised levator muscle, effectively reducing the incidence of CRM positivity (Figure 3.3b). The prone jack-knife position affords excellent views during the

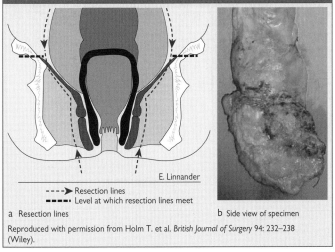

Figure 3.3 Abdominoperineal resection by the extended posterior perineal approach. a Dissections from above and below meet at the top of the levator muscle; b this leaves the levator attached to the mesorectum, which creates a 'cylindrical' specimen

E. Linnander

- - - -▶ Resection lines
■ ■ ■ ■ ■ Level at which resection lines meet

a Resection lines

b Side view of specimen

Reproduced with permission from Holm T. et al. *British Journal of Surgery* 94: 232–238 (Wiley).

perineal dissection; this in turn reduces the chances of entering the wrong surgical plane and perforating the specimen. The superior quality of the resection specimen following a 'cylindrical' resection was demonstrated in a joint UK (Leeds) and Swedish (Stockholm) study. This showed CRM involvement rates of 14.8% vs. 40.6% and intra-operative perforation rates of 3.7% vs. 22.8% in the 'cylindrical' and standard abdominoperineal groups respectively.

Suggested reading

Guidelines for the Management of Colorectal Cancer, The Association of Coloproctology of Great Britain and Ireland, 3rd edition, 2007.

Holm T, Ljung A, Haggmerk T, Jurell G, Lagergren J (2007) Extended abdomino-perineal resection with gluteus maximus flap reconstruction of the pelvic floor for rectal cancer. *British Journal of Surgery* **94**(2): 232–8.

Jayne DG, Guillou PJ, Thorpe H, Quirke P (2007) Randomized trial of laparoscopic-assisted resection of colorectal carcinoma: 3-year results of the UK MRC CLASICC Trial Group. *J Clin Oncol* **25**(21): 3061–8.

Kapiteijn E, Marijnen CA, Nagtegall ID (2001) Preoperative radiotherapy combined with total mesorectal excision for resectable rectal cancer. *N Engl J Med* **345**(9): 638–46.

Sargent N (2001) Refining Multimodal therapy for rectal cancer. N *Engl J Med* **345**: 690–2.

Chapter 4

Radiotherapy and rectal cancer

Rachel Cooper and Paul Hatfield

Key points

- In addition to important surgical advances in the management of rectal cancer, radiotherapy plays a key role in the multidisciplinary management of this disease in selected patients
- There is now an extensive evidence base supporting its role in the neoadjuvant and adjuvant setting
- Radiotherapy is a valuable method of palliation in patients with uncontrolled pelvic disease
- In some patients, with very early disease, radiotherapy can sometimes be used as an alternative to conventional surgery
- Radiotherapists should work closely with other members of the rectal cancer team to ensure that all appropriate patients are offered the benefits of radiotherapy throughout the course of their disease.

4.1 Indications

The main uses of radiotherapy in rectal cancer are:

- Reducing the risk of local recurrence after resection of rectal cancer
- Treating locally advanced disease (often with chemotherapy) to allow an attempt at curative surgery
- Potentially converting a planned abdomino-perineal resection (APR) into an anterior resection (i.e. sphincter preservation)
- Alternative radical treatment for those with early cancers who are either too unfit or unwilling to have surgery
- Palliation.

4.2 **Reducing the risk of recurrence in resectable disease**

When patients are diagnosed with rectal cancer they should be staged as accurately as possible to allow the most appropriate treatment to be planned. The presence or absence of metastases is usually determined with a computed tomography (CT) scan of chest, abdomen and pelvis. Magnetic resonance imaging (MRI) of the pelvis is considered the gold-standard for local staging of the rectal primary. However, in very early disease, endo-rectal ultrasound (ERUS) is better at determining the depth of invasion within the muscle wall of the rectum.

The resectability of the tumour by total mesorectal excision (TME) is determined by assessing the proximity of the tumour to the mesorectal fascia (the planned circumferential resection margin—CRM—in a TME). This would include the primary tumour and any clearly involved mesorectal lymph nodes. Those tumours that are >1–2 mm from the CRM are considered resectable. Some tumours within this group will be at higher risk for local recurrence after surgery than others. For instance, those with significant T3 extension into mesorectal fat, involved mesorectal nodes or extra-mural vascular invasion would fall into this group. Lower third tumours, requiring APR, could also be considered high risk in view of the anatomical challenges of achieving complete resection and the higher risk of spread to pelvic side-wall nodes.

As will be discussed, radiotherapy has been shown to significantly reduce the risk of local recurrence after surgery. The relative risk reduction appears very similar in all patient groups. However, there is controversy about what proportion of the patients in the resectable group should be offered radiotherapy since the 'number needed to treat' to prevent one recurrence will be less if treatment is targeted at the higher risk patients and considerably more if all resectable patients are treated (see Table 4.1). Given that radiotherapy is known to have both acute and delayed toxicity, this decision requires clinical judgement and ideally patient participation.

The evidence base demonstrating that adjuvant radiotherapy reduces local recurrence after surgery is very strong. A meta-analysis of 22 randomised trials using pre or post-operative radiotherapy regimes, published in 2001, demonstrated this convincingly. It also suggested that pre-operative techniques, especially those with higher biologically effective doses (BEDs), were superior. Subsequent analyses of pre-operative radiotherapy from other groups have come to similar conclusions.

Many of the studies evaluated in these overviews came from an era before the introduction of modern TME surgery (which, by resecting the whole mesorectum, reduces the risk of an involved CRM).

Table 4.1 Local recurrence rates related to initial stage of disease in a large, multicentre, randomized trial assessing the role of radiotherapy in rectal cancer (comparing routine SCPRT and selective post-operative CRT for patients with an involved CRM)

TNM Stage	3-year local recurrence (routine SCPRT)	3-year local recurrence (selective post-operative CRT)	Absolute risk reduction	Number needed to treat (to prevent one recurrence at 3 years)
I	1.9%	2.8%	0.9%	111
II	1.9%	6.4%	4.5%	22
III	7.4%	15.4%	8%	13

Table based on data from Sebag-Montefiore, *The Lancet* 2009.

There seems little doubt that this advance alone has significantly reduced the risk of local recurrence. There are clear theoretical reasons to expect this, given the importance of an involved CRM in predicting local recurrence, and a range of clinical datasets confirms it. It could therefore be argued that radiotherapy in these early trials was merely compensating for inadequate surgery. However, two large randomized clinical trials where TME was used, comparing short-course pre-operative radiotherapy (SCPRT—see below) with selective post-operative strategies, have continued to show a benefit from radiotherapy.

Radiotherapy can be given in a variety of ways. 'Conventional', 'long-course' fractionated treatment divides a total dose of 45–50.4 Gy into daily fractions of 1.8–2 Gy, given 5 days a week over 5–6 weeks. In many parts of the world this has been the standard approach in rectal cancer. In Northern Europe, on the other hand, the use of pre-operative radiotherapy was approached cautiously, with a desire not to delay definitive surgical treatment excessively. This lead to the use of a 'short-course' treatment, with 25 Gy given in 5 fractions of 5 Gy over one week (SCPRT), followed by surgery within 7–10 days. Biologically this has a similar effect to the longer regimes, although theoretically there could be higher rates of late toxicity. Long-course treatments have often been given with chemotherapy. This, combined with the extra visits for the patient to the radiotherapy centre, increases cost, time and inconvenience.

Randomized trials show that both approaches are effective at reducing local recurrence and there is, as yet, no convincing evidence that one approach is better than the other. In the case of long-course treatment, the addition of concurrent chemotherapy (chemoradiotherapy—CRT) improves efficacy and a pre-operative approach is superior to a post-operative one.

4.3 **Treating locally advanced disease to achieve curative resection**

The definition of 'locally advanced disease' has been applied to a spectrum of disease that ranges from resectable T3N1 on ERUS to fixed tumours invading neighbouring organs. More recently, pelvic MRI has allowed the identification of patients where primary resection is likely to result in an involved CRM (either macro- or microscopically). However, despite the lack of a consistent definition, there is general agreement that this group of patients should receive pre-operative CRT, despite only limited randomized trial evidence.

Commonly, CRT involves the use of 5-fluorouracil (5-FU) given by continuous infusion, short daily infusions with leucovorin or as the oral pro-drug capecitabine. There have been a number of non-randomized phase II trials and retrospective reviews examining the role of two or more drugs in combination with radiotherapy for locally advanced disease. In general these have reported a higher number of complete responses and promising rates of margin-negative resection and local control. However, until recently, there have been no randomized trials comparing standard CRT with multi-drug regimes. Interestingly, preliminary results from two trials comparing oxaliplatin/5-FU with 5-FU alone have not shown improved outcomes despite increased toxicity. In the UK this has led to interest in a randomized comparison of standard CRT with or without irinotecan.

Some patients with locally advanced disease are not suitable for CRT due to impaired performance status or co-morbidities. For these patients, SCPRT followed by an elective delay of 6–8 weeks (to allow maximal tumour response) can be a useful alternative.

4.4 **Sphincter-preservation**

With improvements in surgical technique it has become possible to perform more sphincter preserving surgery (SPS) in patients with low lying rectal tumours. However, many surgeons believe that low lying tumours (3–6 cms from the anal verge) always require an abdomino-perineal excision of rectum (APER), particularly if the sphincter is invaded. In addition, SPS may not be possible in bulky anterior tumours within a narrow pelvis.

It has been controversial whether the use of pre-operative radiotherapy or CRT can convert a planned APER into a safe low anterior resection, without adversely affecting outcome. A systematic review of randomized trials addressing this issue concluded that it could not but this continues to be debated. What does seem to be clear is that successful SPS depends significantly on the skill and experience of the surgeon.

4.5 **High dose radiotherapy alone**

Radical surgery with or without (neo)adjuvant (chemo)radiotherapy remains the standard of care in rectal cancer. However, there are a small group of patients with early rectal cancer who do not have conventional surgery, either due to co-morbidity or because they choose not to expose themselves to the risks/consequences. High dose radiotherapy alone might be an option for this group of patients. Currently, the most commonly used method is 'contact therapy' which involves the use of superficial x-rays to treat the primary tumour (often combined with external beam chemoradiotherapy to treat the nodes). Some patients are also treated by local excision, using transanal endoscopic microsurgery (TEM) prior to this therapy. There have been no randomized trials, but single centre case series describe local failure rates of 10–20% in T1/T2 tumours.

4.6 **Palliation**

For patients with uncontrolled pelvic disease, radiotherapy remains an important palliative treatment. Symptoms such as pain, bleeding and discharge respond particularly well, although the maximal response can take several weeks to achieve. Obstructive symptoms or diarrhoea respond less well and may be better managed by defunctioning or stenting.

4.7 **Toxicity of radiotherapy**

Following surgery for rectal cancer, patients may experience increased bowel frequency, incontinence (up to 50% will experience some dysfunction and in approximately 15% it will be severe) and sexual dysfunction (erectile and ejaculatory problems in men, severe in 15%; vaginal dryness and dyspareunia in women, severe in 10%). Evidence from randomised trials suggests that radiotherapy increases these risks. Radiotherapy will also produce infertility and increase the risk of late small bowel obstruction (reported in approximately 11% of patients).

Radiotherapy toxicity is reduced by using a pre-operative rather than a post-operative approach. Technique is also important, with smaller volumes producing less normal tissue complications. Modern radiotherapy planning allows the target volume to be more precisely defined. The dose to organs at risk can also be calculated more accurately. By shaping the irradiated volume to the target volume as much as possible this can be minimized.

Studies of SCPRT have described a small increase in the risk of femoral neck and pelvic fractures, especially in the first few years.

By comparison, there is very little published information on the late toxicity after pre-operative CRT. A small randomized study from Poland (comparing rates of SPS after SCPRT or CRT) identified no significant difference in long term toxicity between the two arms. This suggests that despite the concern about the high dose per fraction of SCPRT causing more late toxicity, there is little data to support this view at present.

4.8 **Conclusions**

Radiotherapy is a valuable method for reducing the risk of local recurrence after rectal cancer surgery. A pre-operative approach is generally less toxic and more effective. In resectable disease, SCPRT appears a useful strategy and may be most appropriate when targeted at patients with the highest risk of recurrence. In patients with tumours that are predicted to be unresectable at presentation, pre-operative CRT is the standard approach, giving the best chance for successful down-staging of the tumour (Figure 4.1). Radiotherapy should be considered for the palliation of uncontrolled pelvic disease.

Figure 4.1 **A proposed treatment algorithm for potentially resectable rectal cancer. EMVI = extra-mural vascular invasion, CRT = chemoradiotherapy, SCPRT = short-course pre-operative radiotherapy (usually followed by surgery within 7–10 days), CRM = circumferential resection margin visualized on MRI**

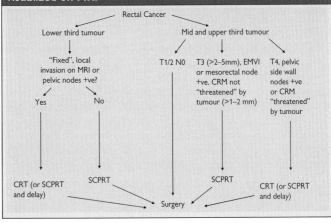

Suggested reading

Adjuvant radiotherapy for rectal cancer: a systematic overview of 8,507 patients from 22 randomised trials (2001) *Lancet* **358**(9290): 1291–1304.

Bosset, J. F., G. Calais, et al. (2005) Enhanced tumorocidal effect of chemotherapy with preoperative radiotherapy for rectal cancer: preliminary results—EORTC 22921. *J Clin Oncol* **23**(24): 5620–7.

Bujko, K., L. Kepka, et al. (2006) Does rectal cancer shrinkage induced by preoperative radio(chemo)therapy increase the likelihood of anterior resection? A systematic review of randomised trials. *Radiother Oncol* **80**(1): 4–12.

Gerard, J. P., T. Conroy, et al. (2006) Preoperative radiotherapy with or without concurrent fluorouracil and leucovorin in T3-4 rectal cancers: results of FFCD 9203. *J Clin Oncol* **24**(28): 4620–5.

Kapiteijn, E., C.A. Marijnen, et al. (2001) Preoperative radiotherapy combined with total mesorectal excision for resectable rectal cancer. *N Engl J Med* **345**(9): 638–46.

Sauer, R., H. Becker, et al. (2004) Preoperative versus postoperative chemoradiotherapy for rectal cancer. *N Engl J Med* **351**(17): 1731–40.

Sebag-Montefiore, D., R.J. Stephens, et al. (2009) Preoperative radiotherapy versus selective postoperative chemoradiotherapy in patients with rectal cancer (MRC CR07 and NCIC-CTG C016): a multicentre, randomised trial. *Lancet* **373**(9666): 811–20.

Sun Myint, A., R. J. Grieve, et al. (2007) Combined modality treatment of early rectal cancer: the UK experience. *Clin Oncol (R Coll Radiol)* **19**(9): 674–81.

Chapter 5

Pharmacology of anti-cancer drugs

Luis Daverede and Daniel Swinson

Key points

- Fluorouracil (5FU) is an anti-metabolite that was rationally synthesised in the 1960s. The reduction of the pyrimidine ring by dihydropyrimidine dehydrogenase, widely expressed in tissues through out the body, is the rate limiting step dehydrogenase (DPD). Five percent of patients are DPD deficient and experience disproportionate toxicity

- Capecitabine, tegafur and S-1 are oral prodrugs which are metabolised to 5FU and other metabolites. The first 2 have at least equal efficacy but better toxicity profiles than bolus 5FU regimens

- Oxaliplatin is a member of the platinum family, that although has no recognised single agent activity has synergy with fluoropyrimidines against colorectal cancer. Cumulative neurotoxicity is the dose limiting toxicity

- Irinotecan is a topoisomerase I inhibitor with both single agent activity and synergy with fluoropyrimidines against colorectal cancer. Aggressive early use of loperamide is important to prevent profuse diarrhoea

- Bevacizumab, cetuximab and panitunumab are monoclonal antibodies, the former targets the vascular endothelial growth factor (VEGF) and is only active in combination with chemotherapy, the latter 2 target epidermal growth factor receptor (EGFR) and have single agent activity and at least an additive effect with chemotherapy against colorectal cancer.

5.1 Fluoropyrimidines

5.1.1 Fluorouracil

Fluorouracil (5-FU) is widely used in solid tumour oncology and forms the backbone of systemic therapy for colorectal cancer. Over the past two decades pro-drugs, capecitabine and tegafur + UFT have been designed to enable oral administration.

5.1.1.1 Mechanism of action

Active metabolites of 5-FU

- are incorporated into RNA and interfere with its synthesis and function
- are incorporated into DNA and affect its stability
- form a ternary complex with thymine synthetase (TS) that is stabilised by reduced folate. This complex inhibits TS function so interfering with DNA synthesis, repair resulting in DNA strand breaks.

The mode of action of 5-FU varies between different tissues, tumours and by administration schedules. Preclinical experiments suggest short exposure to high drug levels induces TS inhibition and longer exposure to lower levels effects RNA function. In practice bolus and infusional regimens are often combined in the commonly used de Gramont (dG) and modified de Gramont (MdG) schedules to take advantage of both modes of action.

5.1.1.2 Mechanism of elimination

Over 90% of 5-FU, administered by bolus injection and virtually all delivered by continuous infusion is eliminated by catabolism. Renal excretion has a lesser but important role. The rate limiting step is reduction of the pyrimidine ring by dihydropyrimidine dehydrogenase (DPD). The highest levels of this enzyme are in hepatocytes but it is also expressed in other cell types, especially in the gastrointestinal mucosa and peripheral lymphocytes. Its activity is saturable hence clearance deviates from a linear relationship at high levels and toxicity becomes unpredictable. DPD levels are deficient in ~5% of patients leading to increased early toxicity and disproportionate myelosuppression. The major metabolite is fluoro-β-alanine (FBAL) that contributes to 5-FU related toxicity and is excreted in the urine.

Oral ftorafur has been combined uracil (DPD inhibitor) as UFT and LV and is delivered in three daily doses. With a 28 day schedule this regimen was found to be better tolerated than twice or once daily dosing.

5.1.1.3 Toxicity of 5-FU by schedule

The dose limiting toxicities for bolus schedules are mucositis and diarrhoea and for infusional schedules is mucositis although diarrhoea still occurs to a lesser extent. Myelosuppression is more problematic with bolus schedules and plantar palmar erythrodysesthesia (hand foot syndrome) is more problematic with infusional schedules.

Mucositis can occur throughout the GI tract and cause dysphagia, retrosternal pain, nausea, abdominal pain, watery diarrhoea and proctitis. Less common serious toxicities include acute neurotoxicity characterized by cerebellar dysfunction and cardiac toxicity that manifests as angina. Accepted dogma has attributed the latter to coronary vasospasm but other manifestations include hyper- or hypotension, cardiomyopathy, arrhythmias, conduction disturbances, and cardiac arrest.

Ocular toxicity frequently occurs but is usually mild and limited to increased lacrimation. More significant problems include conjunctivitis and blepharitis that can proceed to tear duct stenosis, ectropion, and keratitis.

5.1.1.4 Key steps that are targeted to enhance efficacy or reduce toxicity

DPD inhibitors have been combined to the oral pro-drug ftorafur to reduce the degradation of 5FU: 5-chloro-2,4-dihydroxypyridine (CDHP) in the S-1 preparation and uracil in UFT. CDHP is a more potent inhibitor than uracil. Orotic acid phosphoribosyl (OPRTase) catalyses the first step of the anabolic pathway resulting in incorporation of fluoruridine triphosphate (FUTP) into RNA in place of uridine triphosphate (UTP). An inhibitor of this enzyme has also been combined with ftorafur to reduce gut toxicity in the S-1 preparation. TS catalyses the transfer of a methyl group from a reduced folate co-factors to the 5' position of deox-uridylate in place of a hydrogen group. The fluorinated state of the 5-FU active metabolite, 5-Fluoro-2'-deoxyuridylate (5-FdUMP) prevents release of this hydrogen and forms an inactive ternary complex with TS. Provision of replete reduced folate pools by co-administration of leucovorin stabilizes this ternary complex and enhances cytotoxicity of 5-FU.

5.1.2 **Oral fluoropyrimidines**

Three oral prodrugs are in common usage, Capecitabine in the West and S-1 in the Far East and UFT worldwide.

Ftorafur (ftorafur-5-FU, FTO, tegafur) is a furan nucleoside that has similar activity to 5-FU with less myelosuppression but more neurotoxicity. Ftorafur is metabolized to 5-FU by 2 pathways. Microsomal cytochrome P-450 initiates one pathway and cytosol thymidine phosphorylase initiates the other. The liver is the major site of P-450 followed by the GI tract. Conversion mostly occurs intracellularly hence plasma concentrations of ftorafur remain higher than 5-FU. Overexpression of tumour thymidine phosphylase (TP) leads to higher tumour levels of 5-FU than in non-malignant tissues. GI toxicities include nausea, mucositis, diarrhoea and cramps. Both intravenous and oral administration schedules have been developed. This regimen is better tolerated than twice or once daily dosing. Two large randomized trials have reported equal activity with bolus 5-FU and less myelosuppression and infection.

Capecitabine is absorbed intact and converted to 5'deoxy-5'-fluorocytidine by carboxylesterase in the liver then to 5'deoxy-5'fluouridine by cytidine deaminase. The final conversion to 5-FU is catalyzed by TP predominatly in tumour cells.

The toxicity profile is similar to bolus 5-FU although grade 3 toxicity is less frequent other than hand-foot syndrome. Single agent capecitabine has not been compared to infusional 5-FU in the general population but studies in combination with oxaliplatin have not shown significant differences in efficacy or toxicity. The FOCUS 2 trial compared capecitabine and MdG as single agents and in combination with oxaliplatin regimens in poor performance and/or elderly patients. Capecitabine was less well tolerated by these frailer patients and caution should be exercised with a low threshold for dose reduction. One prospective case series and individual case reports have suggested that cardiac toxicity is more problematic than with bolus 5-FU regimens.

Capecitabine potentiates the effects of warfarin and other modes of anticoagulation should be considered if necessary.

5.2 **Oxaliplatin**

Amongst all the platinum compounds, oxaliplatin is the only one to have shown particular efficacy against in colon cancer.

5.2.1 **Mechanism of action**
Platinum analogs form covalent binds with purine DNA bases, blocking the normal functions of cellular DNA. Therapeutically active compounds form DNA interstrand adducts as opposed to DNA interstrand cross-links or DNA-platinum-protein cross links. Apoptotic pathways are mediated through mismatch repair genes, p53 and bcl2/bax. DNA damage is also associated with acute, non-apoptotic cell death. A possible explanation of the effectiveness of Oxaliplatin in colorectal cancer, is the relative inability to perform replicative bypass over an oxaliplatin-DNA link as compared with a cisplatin-carboplatin-DNA lesion.

5.2.2 **Toxicity**
The dose limiting toxicity of oxaliplatin is neuropathic characterized by an acute dysaesthesia and/or paraesthesia of the extremities, with or without cramps or laryngopharyngeal dysaesthesia, often triggered by the cold and a chronic peripheral neuropathy. These acute symptoms occur in 95% of patients and usually regress between courses of treatment, although the duration increases with cumulative dose. The chronic peripheral neuropathy becomes more common after a cumulative dose of 480 mg/m^2. When administered with 5FU, the other important toxicities include myelosuppression, diarrhoea, mucositis, and mild to moderate nausea and vomiting. Rare toxicities include anaphylaxis and haemolytic anaemia. There is also emerging data of a risk of exacerbating pre-existing interstitial lung disease.

5.3 Irinotecan

Irinotecan is a Camptothecin derivative which first entered clinical trials in Japan in the 1980s. Camptothecin is a naturally occurring alkaloid found in the Chinese tree Camptotheca acuminata.

5.3.1 Mechanism of action

Irinotecan is a pro-drug and must be first converted by a carboxylesterase-converting enzyme to the active metabolite 7-ethyl-10-hydroxycamptothecin (SN38). SN38 targets DNA Topoisomerase (Topo) I. Topoisomerases are essential enzymes involved in the regulation of DNA topology and are necessary for the preservation of the integrity of the genetic material during DNA metabolism. The main role of Topo I is the relaxation of supercoiled DNA during RNA transcription. SN38 stabilizes the cleavable complex in which Topo I is covalently bound to DNA at a single-stranded break site. DNA damage occurs when a DNA replication fork encounters these cleavable complexes so forming a double strand DNA break.

5.3.2 Toxicity

Common toxicities include nausea and vomiting (86%), fatigue (17%), mucositis (12%), skin toxicity (5%), asthenia, alopecia, and elevated liver transaminases. Febrile neutropaenia occurs in about 3% of patients. The acute cholinergic syndrome (10%) occurs due to rapid and reversible inhibition of acetylcholinesterase by the lactone form of irinotecan and can be induced by co-administration of oxaliplatin. Symptoms may occur shortly or within several hours after drug administration and include diarrhoea, abdominal cramps, nausea, vomiting, diaphoresis, chills, blurred vision, salivation, lacrimation and asymptomatic bradycardia. This syndrome is not life-threatening and responds to subcutaneous atropine. Delayed-onset diarrhoea, occurring after 24 hours, with a peak incidence at day 5 can be life threatening. It is mediated by the metabolite SN38 and irinotecan is contraindicated in patients with inflammatory bowel disease and caution should be used in deficiencies in hepatocellular glucuronidation such as in Gilbert's syndrome. Less common toxicities are pneumonitis, microscopic haematuria, cystitis, dysarthria, and immune thrombocytopaenia.

5.4 Monoclonal antibodies

Monoclonal antibodies target specific proteins involved in the development and progression of cancer. They have the advantage of high specificity. The targets in colorectal cancer are the epidermal growth factor receptor signalling pathway and angiogenesis. Antibodies directed to proteins in both pathways have shown significant activity in the metastatic disease (see Chapter 9).

5.4.1 Cetuximab

Cetuximab is active in patients with Kirsten rat sarcoma (KRAS) wild-type colorectal cancer.

5.4.1.1 Mechanism of action

Cetuximab is a recombinant human/mouse chimeric monoclonal antibody that binds to the human epidermal growth factor receptor (EGFR), preventing the binding of EGF and other ligands. Blocking of the EGFR prevents phosphorylation and activation of tyrosine-kinases related to the receptor, resulting in cell growth inhibition, induction of apoptosis and decreased vascular endothelial growth factor production. EGFR signal transduction results in the GTPase Kirsten rat sarcoma (KRAS) wild-type activation. Tumours with KRAS mutations are not inhibited and may be potentiated by EGFR inhibition.

5.4.1.2 Toxicity

Skin reactions occur in approximately 80% of patients and mainly present as an acneiform rash but can also present as pruritus, dry skin, desquamation, hypertrichosis or paronichia. Skin reactions usually develop within the first 3 weeks of treatment. Other common side effects of cetuximab include infusion-related reactions such as fever, chills, nausea, vomiting, headache, dizziness or dyspnoea that usually occur shortly after the first cetuximab infusion.

5.4.2 Panitumumab

5.4.2.1 Mechanism of action

Panitumumab is a fully human IgG2 antibody that binds to the epidermal growth factor receptor (EGFR), a transmembrane receptor tyrosine kinase of the ErbB (HER) family. Binding of panitumumab to the EGFR inhibits phosphorylation and activation of EGFR-associated kinases, including EGF and transforming growth factor-α, resulting in inhibition of cell growth and decreased production of growth factors such as vascular endothelial growth factor and interleukin-8.

5.4.2.2 Toxicity

The most common adverse events observed were acneiform rash, paronychia, hypomagnesaemia, fatigue, abdominal pain, nausea, diarrhoea, and ocular toxicity. The most serious adverse events reported are infusion reactions, pulmonary fibrosis, severe dermatologic toxicity complicated by infectious sequelae and sepsis.

5.4.3 Bevacizumab

5.4.3.1 Mechanism of action

Bevacizumab is a humanized monoclonal antibody that binds to the vascular endothelial growth factor (VEGF), inhibiting angiogenesis

Drug (metabolite)	Cmax (μg/mL)	Tmax (Hs)	Vd (L)	PPB (%)	t½ (Hs)	Elimination			Clearance
						Liver metabolism	Renal exc.	Other	
5-FU	23.9–534	2	13–18	8–12	0.13–0.23	90%	<10% unchanged	Tissues (DPD)	Variable
Capecitabine	4.67	1.5		<60	0.75	Not significant	3% unchanged 95% (metabolites)	Tissues (DPD)	Variable
5-FU	0.95	2	13–18	10	0.76				
FBAL	5.46	3.34			3.23		50%		
Oxaliplatin	0.86–1.2		149–358	>90	α: 0.28–0.43 β: 16 γ: 273–391	No evidence	54%		222 mL/min
Irinotecan	1.66±0.79		76–157	30–43	5–9.6	Extensive	16% unchanged		47 L/h
SN38	26.3±11.9	1.6–2.8		94	9–11	Glucuronidated	<1%		
Cetuximab	185±55		1.5–6.2	94	70–100	No evidence	No evidence	Intracellular proteolytic catabolism	0.02–0.08 L/h/m²
Bevacizumab	206±60.7		2.4–3.3	97% to VEGF	18–20 days	No evidence	No evidence		0.207 L/day
Panitumumab	213±59				7.5 days	No evidence	No evidence		4.1–4.8mL/day/kg

Shaded rows: drug and metabolites
Abbreviations: dihydropyrimidine dehydrogenase (DPD)

in tumour cells by preventing the effect of VEGF on its receptors (VEGFR-1 and VEGFR-2).

5.4.3.2 Toxicity

Common adverse effects include hypertension, fatigue, abdominal pain and diarrhoea. Uncommon but serious complications include gastrointestinal perforations (possibly higher in the presence of peritoneal disease), fistulae, haemorrhage, and arterial thromboembolism (possibly higher in the elderly and patients with a history of cardiovascular disease). A small increase in the incidence of post-operative haemorrhage or wound healing complications, occurring within 60 days of major surgery, was observed if the patient was being treated with bevacizumab at the time of surgery.

Suggested reading

Chabner. B.A. (2005) *Cancer Chemotherapy and Biotherapy: Principles of Practice.* Lippincott Williams & Wilkins.

Chabot. G.G., et al. (1998) Irinotecan pharmacokinetics. *Bulletin Du Cancer* Spec No: 11–20.

DeVita. V.T. (2008) *Cancer: Principles and practice of Oncology.* Lippincott Williams & Wilkins.

Graham M.A., et al. (2000) Clinical Pharmacokinetics of Oxaliplatin: A Critical Review *Clin Cancer Res* :1205.

Malet-Martino. M., et al. (2002) Clinical Studies of Three Oral Prodrugs of 5-Fluorouracil (Capecitabine, UFT, S-1): A Review. *Oncologist* **7**: 288–323.

Schellens. J.H.M. (2005) *Cancer Clinical Pharmacology.* Oxford University Press.

Chapter 6

Adjuvant chemotherapy

Uschi Hofmann, Fiona Collinson, Peter Hall,
Mike Braun, and Daniel Swinson

Key points

- Adjuvant single agent fluoropyrimidine (Fu) reduces
  the relative risk of death following potentially curative
  surgery by 20–30%. Addition of oxaliplatin reduces
  relative risk by a further 15%
- The risk reduction is proportional to the absolute risk
  so the higher the risk the greater the benefit. Thus
  adjuvant chemotherapy only achieves a meaningful
  benefit for patients with stage III and high risk stage II
  disease
- The benefit from single agent Fu does not diminish
  with age although data is limited for patients over the
  age of 80. In contrast the benefit of the addition of
  oxaliplatin is questionable over the age of 70
- Discussions with patients should include an estimate
  of the chances of benefit with single agent and
  combination adjuvant chemotherapy.

6.1 Introduction

The aim of adjuvant chemotherapy is to reduce the risk of 'relapse'
by eradicating micro metastatic disease prior to progression to incurable disease. This risk increases with stage (see Table 1.3, Chapter 1.)
and reduces with time following surgery. The size of the risk reduction achieved by adjuvant chemotherapy is proportional to the absolute risk. For example single agent Fu will reduce the absolute risk
of relapse for a patient with stage T3N0Mx disease by 4–5% but will
reduce this risk by 17–19% for a patient with stage T3N2Mx disease.

These phenomena are useful in estimating which of 3 potential groups a patient may fall into following surgery:

- Cured—no micrometastatic disease
- Potentially curable—chemo-sensitive micrometastatic disease
- Incurable—chemo-resistant and micrometastatic disease.

Such estimates may form the basis of the clinician/patient discussion concerning the likelihood of benefit of adjuvant chemotherapy.

6.2 **The benefit of adjuvant chemotherapy over observation alone**

Up until the early 1980s randomized controlled trials (RCT) failed to demonstrate an overall survival (OS) benefit for adjuvant 5-fluorouracil (5-FU) chemotherapy. The 1st RCT to report a significant OS benefit was the National Surgical Adjuvant Breast and Bowel Project (NSABP) C-01 where a survival benefit was seen for lomustine, vincristine and 5-FU (MOF) chemotherapy at 5 years although was lost with longer follow up.

In the mid to late 1980s adjuvant 5-FU was re-evaluated in 2 RCTs in combination with levamisole (LEV), an antihelminthic drug, with immune modulating effects.

- The North Central Cancer Treatment Group (NCCTG) trial included 401 stage II and III patients
- The Eastern cooperative oncology group (ECOG) trial included 1,296 stage II and III patients.

Significant reductions in recurrence rates were seen in both studies. The larger study achieved a significant improvement in OS for patients with stage III but not stage II disease.

On the basis of this evidence, in 1990 a consensus statement by the US National Cancer Institute recommended that 'patients with stage III disease who are unable to enter a clinical trial should be offered adjuvant fluorouracil plus levamisole unless there are medical or psychosocial contraindications.' At this time pre-clinical data was emerging that leucovorin (LV) potentiated the effects of 5-FU by stabilizing the binding to thymidylate synthetase thereby extending enzyme inhibition (Ch 5). Five contemporaneous trials combined different doses of LV with 5-FU.

- The NSABP C-03 trial confirmed superiority of 5-FU and high dose LV over MOF chemotherapy
- The NCCTG group conducted a further study against observation with 6 cycles of 5-FU (425 mg/m^2) with low dose LV (20 mg) given days 1–5, every 4–5 weeks (the 'Mayo clinic' regimen) and found a significant improvement in relapse free and OS

- The position of 5-FU/ LV as a standard of care was further strengthened by the IMPACT (International Multicentre Pooled Analysis of Colon Cancer Trials) report from three parallel trials of 5-FU/ LV against observation with an *a priori* agreement for a pooled analysis when there were sufficient events to prove at least 10% difference in OS. This was achieved with 1,526 patients randomized, the risk of death was reduced by 22% and events by 35%. Subgroup analysis again suggested the benefit was restricted to patients with node positive disease.

6.2.1 Dose of LV and use of levamisole

Subsequent studies compared the addition of different doses of LV versus or in combination with LEV to 5-FU. None of these strategies conferred a benefit. In the largest study, the Quick And Simple And Reliable (QUASAR) trial, the combination was found to be detrimental. A concerning association with multifocal cerebral de-myelinating syndrome caused LEV to fall further from favour.

6.2.2 Duration of treatment

Two large studies found no benefit in continuing treatment beyond 6–8 months.

- The US Intergroup (INT) 0089 trial recruited 3,794 patients, the experimental treatment consisted of the Mayo clinic regimen or weekly 5-FU and high dose LV for 6 weeks with 2 weeks off [the Roswell Park (RPMI) regimen] or the low dose LV plus LEV (LDLV plus LEV) and 5-FU regimen for 30–32 weeks and the control arm was 12 months of 5-FU/LEV
- A collaborative trial of the NCCTG and National Cancer Institute of Canadian trials recruited 915 patients and compared 5-FU and levamisole with the addition of LV for either 6 or 12 months.

A third smaller German study found a similar result. The UK SAFFA trial even suggested that 3 months of infusional 5-FU was sufficient but the study was underpowered and has not changed practice.

6.2.3 Scheduling of 5-FU

Toxicity of 5-FU has been found to be schedule dependent.

- This was clearly demonstrated by the INT 0089 trial where the Mayo clinic regimen was more toxic especially with regard to diarrhoea, in women compared to men and in older patients. This was also seen in a retrospective analysis of the QUASAR trial.
- In the advanced setting infusional 5-FU was shown to be superior to bolus regimens in terms of toxicity and to a lesser extent efficacy.
- Four studies have compared the Mayo clinic regimen with infusional regimens in the adjuvant setting. Similar benefits in terms

of toxicities but not efficacy have been found and therefore have not justified the placement of a central venous catheter necessary for infusional regimens.

6.2.4 **Oral fluoropyrimidines**

The bioavailability of oral 5-FU is erratic due to variance in the expression of dihydropyrimidine dehydrogenase (DPD) in the GI tract. Capecitabine and UFT/Uracil are oral prodrugs of 5-FU that have replaced bolus 5-FU regimens in the advanced setting. Two RCT involving the capecitabine or UFT/Uracil pro-drugs have been conducted.

- The X-ACT trial randomized 1987 stage III colon cancer patients to either capecitabine (1,250 mg/m^2 administered twice daily on days 1–14 every 3 weeks) or the Mayo clinic regimen and was powered to prove equivalence in terms of disease free survival (DFS). Capecitabine was at least equivalent to the Mayo regimen, in terms of DFS [hazard ratio (HR) = 0.87, 0.75–1.00 P<0.001] and OS (HR = 0.84, 0.69–1.01 P<0.001), with reduced toxicity; lower rates of stomatitis, nausea and vomiting, alopecia, diarrhoea and neutropenia but higher rates of hand foot syndrome (HFS) and hyperbilirubinaemia. The latter, with otherwise normal liver function is often due to haemolysis and not clinically relevant. Whilst capecitabine appeared tolerable, dose reductions were necessary in 50% of patients

- The NSABP trial C-06 randomized 1608 patients with resected stage II or III colon cancer to bolus weekly 5-FU/ high-dose LV or UFT/ oral LV. No difference was seen in terms of DFS (HR = 1.004; 95% CI, 0.847 to 1.190) and OS (HR = 1.014; 95% CI, 0.825 to 1.246) and the toxicity profiles, including rates of HFS were comparable. The trial employed a three times daily UFT/ LV dosing regimen, which has raised concerns with compliance and limited use in routine UK practice. Where HFS is problematic UFT/ LV maybe a useful alternative to capecitabine.

6.3 **Combination chemotherapy**

Both oxaliplatin and irinotecan in combination with 5-FU/LV are effective and approved for the treatment of metastatic colorectal cancer.

Three RCTs, have established a role for oxaliplatin in the adjuvant setting.

- The MOSAIC (Multi-center international study of oxaliplatin/5-FU/ leucovorin in the adjuvant treatment of colon cancer) trial randomized 2,246 patients with stage II or III colon cancer to oxaliplatin 85 mg/m^2 day 1, 200 mg/m^2 LV, 5-FU 400 mg/m^2

followed by 2,200 mg/m^2 22-hour infusion days 1 and 2 (FOLFOX) or the 5-FU regimen alone (LV5-FU2). After a median of 38 months follow up the 3 year DFS was improved from 81 to 86% (HR = 0.77; 95% CI 0.65 to 0.91; P = 0.002). No survival benefit was reported at time of publication in 2004. An update on DFS after median follow up of 82 months revealed a durable improvement with 5 year DFS rates of 73% versus 67% (HR, 0.80; P = 0.003) and 6 year OS rates 78% versus 76.0%, respectively (HR = 0.84; P = 0.046). Subgroup analysis suggested the absolute benefit in stage II disease was very modest. Furthermore the OS benefit even in N1 disease is likely to be less than 5% in the majority of patients.

- The NSABP C-07 (National Surgical Adjuvant Breast and Bowel Project C-07) study randomly assigned 2,492 patients to receive the RPMI regimen alone or in combination with oxaliplatin (FLOX). After a median follow up of 42.5 months the results were near identical to the MOSAIC trial, the 4 year DFS rates were 67.3% and 73.2% respectively (HR = 0.80; log-rank P = 0.004). More mature data with a median follow up of 84.5 months has shown a persistent DFS benefit at 7 years but no OS benefit has yet emerged

- The substitution of infusional 5-FU with capecitabine was investigated in the NO16968 trial. The study randomized 1886 patients to capecitabine 1250 mg/m^2 and oxaliplatin 130 mg/m^2 (XELOX) or the Mayo clinic regimen for 6 months. After a median follow-up of 57 months, an analysis again found near identical efficacy results to the MOSAIC trial with significantly superior DFS for XELOX (71.0 vs. 67.0%, HR 0.80, P=0.0045). Interim OS results find no benefit yet.

Cumulative dosing of oxaliplatin beyond 6 cycles commonly results in a chronic peripheral neuropathy. Over 10% of patients will suffer a grade 3 neuropathy which may persist at this severity for over a year in 1% of patients. As this effect can deteriorate even after stopping oxaliplatin there should be a low threshold for stopping oxaliplatin after six cycles.

Irinotecan's potential in the adjuvant setting has been investigated by 2 RCTs recruiting over 3,500 patients but in contrast to oxaliplatin no benefit has been observed.

- The Pan-European Trials in Adjuvant Colon Cancer (PETACC)-3 and Federation Nationale des Centres de Lutte contre le (FNCLCC) Accord02 trials used the same control arm as the MOSAIC trial and combined this with fortnightly irinotecan. Disappointingly, no benefit in DFS or OS was seen and increased toxicity was seen in the study arms

- The CALGB 89803 trial evaluated the addition of irinotecan to bolus 5-FU/LV and also found no benefit.

A strong association between improvement in 3-year disease free survival and consequent improvements in 5 year OS has been reported by Sargent et al. This has led to the approval of FOLFOX by the US Food and Drug Administration (FDA) as standard adjuvant treatment for stage III colon cancer after a curative resection. Irinotecan remains reserved for patients with advanced disease.

6.4 Biological agents

In many countries the monoclonal antibodies, bevacizumab and cetuximab that target the vascular endothelial growth factor (VEGF) and the epidermal growth factor receptor (EGFR), respectively, are well established in the treatment of advanced disease. To date studies in the adjuvant setting have been disappointing.

- The NSABP C-08 trial compared FOLFOX chemotherapy with FOLFOX/Bevacizumab. Despite improving 1 year DFS, no benefit was seen at 3 years
- The NCCTG INT N0147 trial compared FOLFOX with or without cetuximab. No benefit in 3 year DFS was found
- The AVANT study has a similar design but included a XELOX plus bevacizumab arm. No formal results have been presented yet but a provisional report was been released in late 2010 that suggested that there may be a detrimental effect of adding bevacizumab to combination adjuvant chemotherapy. The QUASAR 2 study that was randomizing patients to capecitabine and bevacizumab or capecitabine alone was subsequently stopped and bevacizumab withdrawn from patients randomised to the experimental arm.

6.5 Management of specific groups

6.5.1 Stage II disease

The role of adjuvant chemotherapy for patients with stage II disease remains controversial. Subgroup analyses of individual studies and meta-analyses have suggested only a borderline benefit for adjuvant chemotherapy in this group although one large trial has provided firmer supportive evidence.

- The IMPACT B2 study (International Multicentre Pooled Analysis of B2 Colon Cancer Trials) included 1,016 stage II patients and reported a 2% non-statistically significant difference in 5-year OS
- In the QUASAR trial uncertain arm investigators were invited to randomize patients that they were unsure would benefit from adjuvant chemotherapy to single agent 5-FU or observation.

A significant OS benefit of 3.8% was reported following recruitment of 3,238 (91% stage II) patients. However when just stage II disease was analysed no significant benefit was seen.

There has been an acceptance that a trial of sufficient size (4,800 patients) to answer this question is unlikely to be undertaken. In view of the consistency of relative risk reduction across different stages a pragmatic approach has been adopted. Selected patients with high risk stage II cancers are routinely offered single agent Fu chemotherapy.

- The ASCO guidelines include T4, low nodal yield (<12), high histological grade, extramural vascular invasion, acute obstruction and tumour perforation at presentation as markers of high risk.

These prognostic markers help inform the discussion concerning future events but are not necessarily predictive of benefit from chemotherapy. Sadly we lack robust predictive markers in planning adjuvant chemotherapy but there are potential candidates.

- 18q loss of heterozgosity (LOH) is a marker of chromosomal instability and poor prognosis. Some retrospective studies have found an association with lack of response to Fu chemotherapy. Overall results are inconsistent and methological concerns have been raised relating to the variety of 18q markers used, degree of micro dissection of tumours and quality control used. Further prospective studies are needed

- Microsatellite instability (MSI) occurs due to defects in the mismatch repair process and is seen in patients with Lynch syndrome and also some sporadic cancers (see Chapter 1). Tumours are classed as MSI-high (H), MSI-low (L) or microsatellite stable (MSS) depending on the presence or absence and frequency of these defects. Ribic et al. conducted a retrospective analysis of 1,027 tumour samples from seven RCT with observation only arms. The association between MSI status, stage of disease and degree of benefit from adjuvant chemotherapy was studied. In the untreated population MSI-H was associated with a better prognosis but this was lost with the use of adjuvant chemotherapy. Subgroup analysis of the MSI-H patients suggested that patients with stage II disease faired worse with adjuvant chemotherapy (102 patients) and those with stage III disease derived no benefit (63 patients). Conversely in MSS patients (428 stage II and 434 stage III patients) the effects of adjuvant chemotherapy were consistent with the expected benefit. Whilst this data is compelling the numbers are small and the analysis is retrospective. Analysis has also been conducted in the QUASAR uncertain arm where patients were also randomized between chemotherapy and observation. MSI was again found to be a good prognostic factor but was not found to be a significant predictive marker.

MSI status has been approved by the FDA as a predictive markers for patients with stage II disease although has not been widely used in the UK. In view of the good prognosis of MSI-H stage II disease the absolute benefit of adjuvant chemotherapy is likely to be of doubtful clinical significance.

• Further data will be available from the Intergroup study E5202 that is enrolling patients with MSS and no 18q LOH or MSI-H to an observation only strategy.

6.5.2 The elderly

The median age of patients participating in published RCTs of adjuvant chemotherapy is in the low 60s where as the median age for patients diagnosed with colorectal cancer is over the age of 70. Data from studies of full dose single agent Fu in the elderly have reported high levels of toxicity especially over the age of 80. Nevertheless over 40% of patients over the age of 75 may be deemed fit for chemo-therapy on the basis of performance status alone and often have a life expectancy of greater than 10 years. Pooled analysis from older trials and a subgroup analysis of the X-ACT study support the use of adjuvant single agent Fu in selected elderly patients. The use of combination chemotherapy in this population appears less justified.

• A pooled analysis from seven RCT trials, involving 3,351 patients, comparing adjuvant 5-FU based regimens with observation found no diminished benefit in the elderly patients (>70 years of age) although the survival curves started to converge after 5 years. Leucopenia was the sole toxicity index that was increased. Only 0.7% of patients were over the age of 80 and so caution is still recommended for octogenarians

• Further supportive evidence has been obtained from an analysis 4,768 Medicare patients aged ≥65 and from data from the National Cancer Data Base in the US that suggests the magnitude of benefit is similar to that seen in younger patients

• A subgroup analyses of the MOSAIC and the NSABP C-07 trials found no additional benefit for the addition of oxaliplatin for elderly patients. A meta-analysis of the irinotecan studies, these 2 oxaliplatin studies and the X-ACT trial found the additional ben-efit of 'modern' chemotherapy was limited to patients under the age of 70. This analysis has been criticized for including one trial designed to show equivalence and two negative trials. A meta-analysis of the three positive oxaliplatin trials is awaited.

6.6 Health economics

In financially constrained healthcare systems new interventions must be cost-effective if they are to be adopted. Canada and Australia were among the first to consider cost-effectiveness explicitly in the drug approval process. A framework used by many countries for determining cost-effectiveness relies on the cost per quality adjusted life-year (QALY) gained. A QALY is a unit of measurement for health-gain where improvement in life-expectancy is waited for quality. In the United Kingdom the National Institute for Health and Clinical Excellence (NICE) was introduced in 1999 with the objective of providing equitable access to healthcare across the country. It has used this framework to dictate which drugs the NHS should pay for. On this basis, in the adjuvant setting, capecitabine is thought to be a cost-effective alternative to infusional 5-FU/LV. Drug acquisition costs of capecitabine are currently much higher than 5-FU/LV but cost savings can be made by the avoidance of intravenous administration. Adverse events associated with capecitabine have also been demonstrated to cost less overall. The addition of oxaliplatin to 5-FU/LV has proven to be highly cost-effective in stage III disease although it is less certain whether capecitabine provides value for money over 5-FU/LV when included in combination therapy.

6.7 **Summary**

Adjuvant chemotherapy should be offered to patients following potentially curative surgery with high risk stage II and stage III colorectal cancer. Combination chemotherapy with oxaliplatin and Fu should be considered only for patients with stage III disease. The benefits in most patients with N1 disease are modest and single agent Fu remains a reasonable option for these patients. Increasing age appears to diminish the benefit of combination chemotherapy and should be avoided in the over 70s unless patients are very fit where as it may be considered to a broader population of younger patients. Unfortunately the benefits of VEGF and EGFR targeted therapies in the advanced setting have not been seen in the adjuvant setting and should not be considered.

Suggested reading

Andre. T. et al. (2004) Oxaliplatin, Fluorouracil, and Leucovorin as Adjuvant Treatment for Colon Cancer *N Engl J Med* **350**: 2343.

DeVita. V.T. (2008) *Cancer: Principles and practice of Oncology*. Lippincott Williams & Wilkins.

Gill. S. et al. (2004) Pooled Analysis of Fluorouracil-Based Adjuvant Therapy for Stage II and III Colon Cancer: Who Benefits and by How Much? *J Clin Oncol* **10**: 1797.

Quasar Collaborative Group (2007) Adjuvant chemotherapy versus observation in patients with colorectal cancer: a randomised study *Lancet* **370**: 220.

Sargent D. et al. (2008) Evidence for Cure by Adjuvant Therapy in Colon Cancer: Observations Based on Individual Patient Data From 20,898 Patients on 18 Randomized Trials *J Clin Oncol* **19**: 5632.

Twelves C. et al. (2005) Capecitabine as Adjuvant Treatment for Stage III Colon Cancer *New Engl J Med* **352**: 2696.

Chapter 7

Systemic therapy for advanced colorectal cancer

Fiona Collinson, Peter Hall, Mike Braun, and Daniel Swinson

> **Key points**
> - Over the past two decades the median overall survival for patients with advanced colorectal cancer has increased from 6 months without treatment to 2 years with modern systemic therapies
> - The standard chemotherapy armamentarium includes fluoropyrimidines, oxaliplatin and irinotecan delivered in two lines of treatment. Irinotecan and fluoropyrimidines have single agent activity but oxaliplatin is only effective in combination with a second drug
> - Infusional 5-fluorouracil can be substituted with capecitabine without loss of efficacy. Caution should be exercised in the elderly and in the presence of even modest renal impairment
> - Controversy persists on the worth of newer biological drugs targeting EGFR and VEGF
> - Current research aims to identify new agents and develop a tailored approach dependent on predictive clinicopathological and biological markers.

7.1 Introduction

A third of patients present with advanced disease at initial presentation, and a further quarter relapse following potentially curative treatment. In these settings the treatment of colon and rectal cancer is broadly similar and is considered together in this chapter.

Assuming no potential for curative resection, systemic therapy is usually the primary palliative treatment employed. Active chemotherapy drugs include fluoropyrimidines (5-fluorouracil [5FU] capecitabine and tegafur/uracil (UFT), irinotecan and oxaliplatin. Biological agents include monoclonal antibodies targeting vascular endothelial growth factor (VEGF) (e.g. bevacizumab) and epidermal growth factor receptor (EGFR) (e.g. cetuximab and panitumumab).

The median overall survival (OS) for patients with advanced colorectal cancer has significantly increased over the past 20 years, from 6 months with best supportive care (BSC) alone to around 20–24 months with the use of combination chemotherapy and targeted agents. Recognition must also be given to advances in surgery, supportive care and multidisciplinary team working.

7.2 Study endpoints

The development of end points over and above OS have been necessary in clinical trials due to patients receiving increasing lines of treatment, thereby obscuring the benefit from earlier interventions. Progression free intervals are now frequently used; they are not influenced by subsequent treatments and have been shown to correlate with OS. For trials incorporating planned treatment breaks and/or periods of maintenance therapy other alternatives such as time to strategy failure or duration of disease control have been proposed, although not yet widely adopted.

7.3 Chemotherapy agents

7.3.1 Single-agent fluoropyrimidines

Multiple studies and a subsequent meta-analysis demonstrated 5FU-based chemotherapy improves time to disease progression (TTP), OS and QoL compared to BSC alone (absolute OS benefit 3 to 6 months). Concomitant leucovorin (LV) potentiates the activity of 5FU and improves response rates (RR), whether this equates to any survival improvement is less clear.

Trials conducted in the 1990s explored different 5FU schedules. Infusional 5FU was associated with reduced neutropenia, diarrhoea and mucositis compared to bolus 5FU but requires an indwelling central venous catheter. The 2 most commonly used regimens are the de Gramont (dG) schedule, 2 consecutive days of LV and bolus 5FU followed by a 22 hour 5FU infusion or the modified (M) dG schedule with one LV and bolus 5FU followed by a 46 hour infusion of 5FU delivered fortnightly.

Oral bioavailability of 5FU is poor, predominantly due to significant intra-patient variability of dihydropyrimidine dehydrogenase (DPD) expression (see Chapter 6) in the gastrointestinal tract. Oral pro-drugs have been developed that mimic the pharmacokinetics of infusional 5FU. Capecitabine is the most common used and two RCTs have reported benefits in terms of response rate and toxicity over bolus 5FU regimens. Capecitabine was associated with less stomatitis, alopecia nausea, diarrhoea and neutropenia but more palmar-plantar syndrome. The FOCUS2 study conducted in patients deemed unfit for full dose combination chemotherapy compared capecitabine with infusion 5FU as single agents or in combination with oxaliplatin. No difference in efficacy was seen but capecitabine was associated with increased toxicity. Studies using combination chemotherapy in younger/fitter patients reported similar efficacy and toxicity results. A recent subgroup analysis of the COIN trial that permitted the use of either infusional 5FU or capecitabine suggested differences in toxicity maybe due to renal function; patients with modest impairment in renal function (GFR 50–80) had higher rates of toxicity with capecitabine.

UFT, consists of both tegafur (a 5FU prodrug) and uracil (a competitive inhibitor of DPD). Two randomized phase III studies compared UFT to 5FU and demonstrated no statistical difference in terms of RR, PFS or OS, but less neutropenia and stomatitis in the UFT arms. No direct comparisons with capecitabine or infusional 5FU have been made. Cross trial comparisons suggest reduced palmar-plantar syndrome than capecitabine and more diarrhoea than infusional 5FU.

7.3.2 **Irinotecan**

Irinotecan is a topoisomerase I inhibitor. Initial RCTs reported an OS benefit following progression on single agent 5FU. Subsequently the addition of irinotecan to 1st line 5FU was shown to improve RRs, PFS and OS (Table 7.1). The dose limiting toxicity is diarrhoea, which is more problematic in combination with capecitabine or bolus 5FU than with dG or MdG. The combination of irinotecan and dG or MdG will be abbreviated to FOLFIRI in this chapter.

7.3.3 **Oxaliplatin**

Oxaliplatin is a platinum derivative and its administration is limited by cumulative peripheral sensory neuropathy. As a single agent it has limited activity, but when used in combination with a Fu it has been shown to significantly improve RR and PFS (Table 7.1).

A number of schedules of oxaliplatin combined with dG or MdG have been developed. The standard abbreviation used is FOLFOX with a number to denote which schedule has been used. For simplicity the abbreviation FOLFOX alone will be used in this chapter.

63

Table 7.1 Important RCTs in advanced colorectal cancer

Trial name	Description	Outcome
1st line chemotherapy		
De Gramont et al. 2000	FOLFOX or 5FU	PFS benefit for oxaliplatin
Douillard et al. 2000	FOLFIRI or 5FU	OS benefit for irinotecan
Saltz et al. 2000	FOLFIRI or 5FU or irinotecan alone	OS benefit for combination
N9741	IFL or FOLFOX4	OS benefit for FOLFOX4
FOCUS	Sequential single agent or staged comb or comb	No difference
CAIRO	Staged combination or combination	No difference
COIN	Continuous or intermittent	Unable to prove equivalence
TTD-MACRO	Continuous or intermittent with maintenance Bev	Unable to prove equivalence
2nd line chemotherapy		
Cunningham et al. 1998	BSC +/– line irinotecan	OS benefit for irinotecan
Rothenburg et al.	FOLFOX or 5FU or oxaliplatin alone	PFS benefit for combination
Douillard et al. 2000	FOLFIRI→FOLFOX or FOLFOX→FOLFIRI	No difference
Addition of biologicals		
Hurwitz et al. 2004	IFL +/– Bev	OS benefit for Bev
NO16966	OxFu +/– Bev	PFS benefit for Bev
E3200	FOLFOX +/– Bev	PFS benefit for Bev
CRYSTAL	FOLFIRI +/– Cetux	OS benefit for Cetux
COIN	OxFu +/– Cetux	No difference
PRIME	FOLFOX +/– Pan	PFS benefit for pan
CAIRO2	FOLFOXBev +/– Cetux	PFS harm for Cetux
PACCE	FOLFIRIBev or FOLFOXBev +/– Cetux	PFS harm for Cetux
NORDIC VII	FLOX +/– Cetux	No difference

Abbreviations: FOLFOX: oxaliplatin with fortnightly bolus and infusional 5FU; FOLFIRI: irinotecan with fortnightly bolus and infusional 5FU; FLOX: oxaliplatin with bolus 5FU; IFL: irinotecan with bolus 5FU; cont: continuous; int: intermittent; Cetux: cetuximab; Pan: panitunumab; Bev: bevacizumab.

Oxaliplatin combined with bolus 5FU is referred to as FLOX and when oxaliplatin is combined with capecitabine the abbreviation XELOX has been used. When trials have used either the abbreviation OxFu will be used.

No clear survival advantage has been demonstrated to guide the use of either oxaliplatin or irinotecan based chemotherapy in the 1st line setting. Following progression on 1st line combination chemotherapy clinicians routinely consider the reverse combination. One RCT has suggested a small OS benefit for second line treatment, RRs are low, no higher than 15%, and the chance of controlling disease for more than 6 months is only around 30%. However centres that take an aggressive approach with frequent use of 2nd line chemotherapy have better outcomes.

7.3.4 **Vascular endothelial growth factors (VEGF) inhibitors**

Bevacizumab is chimeric monoclonal antibody that targets VEGF, an important pro-angiogenic agent, and has activity in multiple cancer sites. Common toxicities include reversible hypertension and proteinuria, and less frequently haemorrhage, gastrointestinal perforation and venous and arterial thrombotic events. The latter may occur more commonly with increasing age and coexistent vascular disease. Rarely, reversible posterior leucoencephalopathy, suggested by loss of coordination, confusion, visual loss and headache, has been reported. This is best diagnosed by MRI and features include bilateral white-matter abnormalities suggestive of oedema in the posterior regions of the cerebral hemispheres.

Colorectal cancer was the first disease site where bevacizumab was proven to be an active agent. Three RCTs have studied the addition of bevacizumab to 1st line combination chemotherapy. The 1st, reported by Saltz et al. compared IFL (irinotecan/bolus 5FU) plus bevacizumab to IFL alone and demonstrated a significant improvement in OS in addition to improvements in RR and TTP. However the NO16966 study and a recently published smaller Greek study used oxaliplatin and 5-FU regimens as the chemotherapy backbone and did not confirm benefit from the addition of bevacizumab in terms of OS, PFS or even RR. The results of the Saltz et al. study were further confounded by the N93741 study that found IFL was inferior to FOLFOX suggesting that the control arm of the Saltz study was not optimal. The addition of bevacizumab to single agent Fu chemotherapy has also been addressed by a combined analysis of 2 small randomised studies and a further RCT. A consistent benefit has been demonstrated in terms of PFS and RR.

In the second line setting the E3200 study compared FOLFOX and bevacizumab with either alone. The bevacizumab only arm was stopped early in view of a lack of activity. A significant OS advantage was seen for the FOLFOX and bevacizumab arm although the absolute benefit was modest, 2.1 months.

Taken together these results suggest that bevacizumab is an active drug for the treatment of advanced colorectal cancer although the benefit of its use in the 1st line setting combined with optimal chemotherapy is unclear. In the 1st line setting it maybe better utilised combined with single agent fluoropyrimidines where combination chemotherapy is not feasible or in 2nd line where chemotherapy alone is less effective.

7.3.5 **Epidermal growth factor receptor (EGFR) inhibitors**

The EGFR is a transmembrane protein that initiates an important signalling kinase cascade involved in tumourigenesis (Figure 7.1). Activation stimulates cellular proliferation, angiogenesis and inhibits apoptosis. Panitumumab and cetuximab are monoclonal antibodies (humanized and chimeric respectively) that inhibit EGFR signalling with promising anticancer activity in a number of solid tumours. Common toxicities include rash and diarrhoea.

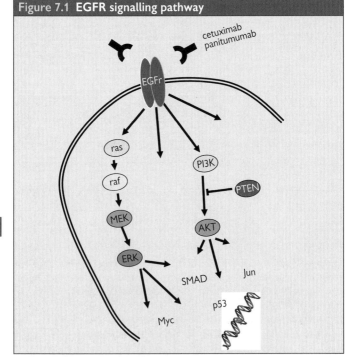

Figure 7.1 EGFR signalling pathway

Interest in cetuximab relating to colorectal cancer was generated with the presentation of the BOND study results. Patients who had progressed on irinotecan were randomised to cetuximab alone or irinotecan/cetuximab. A higher RR was obtained with combination therapy when compared to cetuximab alone, suggesting that cetuximab could re-sensitise patients to irinotecan. Interest was heightened by the BOND2 study, a further randomized phase II trial that reported promising activity for both combined irinotecan, cetuximab, bevacizumab and cetuximab, bevacizumab following progression on second line irinotecan based chemotherapy.

Subsequently two large randomized studies compared these monoclonal antibodies to BSC alone, and found modest benefits in terms of response and PFS. The cetuximab study (C0-17) also reported a small OS benefit. The panitumumab study permitted crossover on progression, which probably masked an OS benefit.

Between 2003 and 2006 the addition of cetuximab to first-line chemotherapy was studied in the CRYSTAL, OPUS, and CAIRO2 trials, to second-line chemotherapy in the EPIC trial. The addition of panitumumab to first-line chemotherapy was studied in the PACCE trial. Fu based chemotherapy was combined with either irinotecan in CRYSTAL or oxaliplatin in OPUS and CAIRO2. EPIC used single agent irinotecan. PACCE used both drugs but analysed the results separately. Bevacizumab was also included as standard in CAIRO2 and PACCE. From 2005 to 2008 the addition of cetuximab to 1st line OxFu was studied in the COIN trial and from 2006 to 2008 the addition of panitumumab to FOLFOX was studied in the PRIME trial and to FLOX in the NORDIC VII trial (Table 7.1).

No study reported a significant OS advantage with the addition of cetuximab although a PFS benefit was seen in CRYSTAL and EPIC. Significant crossover to cetuximab occurred in the control arms of both studies. Both studies that included bevacizumab reported a detrimental effect in the experimental arms, and failed to support the previous results from BOND-2.

Accumulated evidence from single arm studies found mutation (MUT) of Kirsten RAS (KRAS), a signalling kinase down stream of EGFR, predicted resistance to EGFR targeted therapy (Figure 7.1). These mutations are seen in approximately 40% of tumours. Retrospective analysis of the 2 BSC studies confirmed that benefit was confined to patients with wild type (WT) KRAS tumours. A similar picture was seen in the CRYSTAL, EPIC and OPUS trials, with effects on RR especially impressive. The CAIRO2 and PACCE studies found no benefit even in the WT KRAS population. Likewise the COIN and NORDIC VII trials have found no PFS or OS benefit. The PRIME study found a modest a PFS benefit but no improvement in RR and OS analysis is awaited. Pooled analysis from these studies has suggested a harmful effect for EGFR targeted therapies in the MUT KRAS population.

Overall these studies have suggested a modest benefit for the addition of these targeted therapies to 1st line combination chemotherapy. Greater benefit maybe associated with the use of irinotecan and 5FU than with oxaliplatin and capecitabine and these drugs should not be combined with bevacizumab.

7.4 Treatment strategies

7.4.1 Immediate or delayed chemotherapy

One randomized controlled trial (RCT) and a meta-analysis of two other RCTs have compared immediate treatment with a delay until symptoms occur. Both favoured early treatment although the trials in the meta-analysis were stopped early and did not demonstrate a significant survival benefit. These studies were conducted prior to modern day systemic therapies. A cautious watch and wait policy remains an option for patients with low volume asymptomatic disease.

7.4.2 Staged combination chemotherapy

Initial studies reported a consistent benefit for FOLFIRI or FOLFOX over single agent 5FU treatment. However only a minority of patients received second line treatment in these studies as there was no planned cross over following progression. The FOCUS and CAIRO studies sought to explore whether it was safe to start with single agent Fu with an a priori plan to use 2nd line chemotherapy on progression (Table 7.1).

The UK Medical Research Council (MRC) FOCUS study randomized 2,135 patients with advanced, incurable colorectal cancer to arm A, the control arm, of sequential single agent treatment (5FU followed by irinotecan) or arm B, staged combination chemotherapy (5FU followed by FOLFIRI or FOLFOX) or arm C, upfront combination chemotherapy (FOLFIRI or FOLFOX). The primary end point was OS. No significant difference was found between the three approaches although a planned subgroup analysis favoured arm C irinotecan5FU over arm A (median OS 16.7 vs 13.9 months; p = 0.01).

The CAIRO study randomized 820 patients with advanced, incurable colorectal cancer to sequential treatment (capecitabine followed by irinotecan, followed by XELOX) or to combination treatment (capecitabine/irinotecan followed by XELOX). Median OS was 16.3 months in the sequential treatment arm and 17.4 months in the combination treatment arm, demonstrating no statistically significant difference.

The median OS for all arms in both of these studies was lower than expected. In part this can be attributed to the avoidance of patients with potentially operable liver metastases. Additionally a lower than expected proportion of patients were exposed to all three active agents (23% in the FOCUS trial and 36–53% in the CAIRO trial).

Two smaller studies in the UK and France, the LIFE and FFCD 05 trials, respectively reported similar results.

Based on this evidence it is appropriate to consider patients for initial single agent Fu chemotherapy if the treating clinician is confident that the patient will be fit for combination treatment on progression.

The possibility of using all three dugs together upfront has also been considered in two studies with conflicting results. An Hellenic oncology group trial demonstrated no statistically significant benefit for all three drugs in contrast to an Italian study which did demonstrate benefit in terms of PFS and OS. Both studies used a lower 5FU dose in the 5FU/irinotecan arm compared to the three drug arm. A recent systematic review in this field demonstrated a significant benefit in favour of the three drug combination in terms of RR, PFS and OS, at the expense of increased toxicity. This regimen is likely to be most appropriate for young, fit patients with potentially operable disease where maximizing the chance of a significant response is essential.

7.4.3 **Intermittent chemotherapy**
Colorectal cancer differs in some ways from other solid tumour treatments, in that treatments are increasingly being used for defined periods of time, with planned treatment breaks and/or periods of maintenance therapy, followed by re-introduction of previously utilized chemotherapy regimens, potentially combined with alternative drugs which may reintroduce sensitivity. There is no clear consensus in the appropriate duration of chemotherapy. Introducing treatment breaks into chemotherapy scheduling has the advantage of improving quality of life and reducing cost, however evidence is required that this is not detrimental.

A number of different trials have addressed this issue (Table 7.1). The MRC CRO6 study, conducted in the era before combination therapy, investigated continuous single agent 5FU and versus intermittent 5FU with treatment breaks in patients with responding or stable disease at 3 months. OPTIMOX1 looked at FOLFOX until progression or FOLFOX with periods of time off oxaliplatin whilst continuing single agent 5FU. The GISCAD study compared alternating 2 month blocks on and off FOLFIRI treatment with continuous FOLFIRI treatment. OPTIMOX2 subsequently studied FOLFOX with complete treatment breaks compared to FOLFOX with breaks from oxaliplatin alone. The CONcePT study compared FOLFOX bevacizumab with intermittent oxaliplatin with continuous FOLFOX bevacizumab. None of CRO6, OPTIMOX1, GISCAD studies were powered for equivalence. The OPTIMOX2 and CONcePT trials were stopped early for differing reasons. Two trials have been powered for equivalence and completed accrual. The TTD-MACRO study compared XELOX bevacizumab and maintenance bevacizumab with continuous XELOX bevacizumab; the larger MRC COIN trial randomized patients to either continuous OxFu or six cycles of OxFu with rechallenge if the progression free interval was more than 6 weeks.

The initial three studies did not demonstrate any detriment to stopping chemotherapy for a period of time. OPTIMOX2 found a non-significant detrimental effect in the intermittent chemotherapy arm, where as the CONcePT trial suggested the use of intermittent oxaliplatin, was beneficial. However neither TTD-MACRO nor COIN was able to prove non-inferiority for an intermittent chemotherapy approach.

A major concern in many these studies is the failure to re-start chemotherapy as per protocol, this was only achieved in 37%, 55%, and 50% of patients in the CRO6, OPTIMOX-1 and COIN trials, respectively. Patients from centres that routinely complied with re-introduction of oxaliplatin in the OPTIMOX1 trial had better survival than centres that did not, concurring with previous evidence that exposure to all three active chemotherapeutic drugs is essential to maximize survival.

Ongoing trials include the CAIRO 3 trial that is comparing maintenance capecitabine bevacizumab with a complete break following initial XELOX bevacizumab; COIN B has recently completed accrual comparing intermittent FOLFOX with maintenance cetuximab with continuous FOLFOX cetuximab; TTD MACRO02 is comparing continuous FOLFOX cetuximab with FOLFOX cetuximab followed by maintenance cetuximab; finally the DREAM trial is comparing continuous OxFu bevacizumab with OxFu bevacizumab with maintenance bevacizumab erlotinib (a small molecule EGFR tyrosine kinase inhibitor).

7.4.4 **Predictive markers**

Predictive markers are clinicopathological and biological characteristics that are associated with benefit or lack of benefit to a particular therapy.

Tumour KRAS status has already been discussed as a predictive marker for EGFR targeted therapy. BRAF and NRAS are further downstream signalling kinases from EGFR that are also mutated in a proportion of patients and may also predict resistance to EGFR targeted therapies. MUT BRAF and MUT NRAS occur in 6–10% and 1–2% of patients.

One phase II study has suggested serum levels of collagen IV are associated with response to bevacizumab but the predictive power of this marker needs to be confirmed from analysis of samples from a randomised study.

Retrospective biomarker studies from two large RCTs in the UK and Holland have identified potential predictive markers for the benefit of combination over single agent chemotherapy. A benefit for 1st line combination chemotherapy was associated with high Topo I expression in the UK study and low DPD expression in the Dutch study. These data need to be corroborated in further studies.

Subgroup analysis of clinicopathological markers from the COIN study suggests that an initial platelet count over 400 predicts a worse outcome with an intermittent strategy. This has yet to be validated in other studies, biomarker studies are awaited. A similar analysis from the FOCUS trial found a non-significant trend favouring upfront combination chemotherapy in patients with a poor performance status and patients with an initial white cell count over 10.

7.5 **Health economics**

The majority of the chemotherapy agents recommended for routine use in this chapter are currently thought to be cost-effective on the basis of cost per quality adjusted life-year (QALY). Public funding for biological therapies such as bevacizumab and cetuximab has been more controversial, with cost-effectiveness estimates falling far above the historically accepted threshold in many countries. This has been temporarily overcome in some instances by patient access schemes whereby manufacturers subsidize the cost of a drug as part of a complex arrangement. Local or national price negotiations have also played a role. It has become apparent that society may be willing to pay more for treatments in special circumstances such as at the end of life, for rare diseases (including biomarker-selected subgroups) or where treatments are particularly innovative. In the US, the Food and Drug administration is placing increasing emphasis on clinically meaningful endpoints such as overall survival and quality of life rather than surrogate endpoints such as progression-free survival. In 2010 a ring-fenced cancer drug fund was introduced by the UK government, providing temporary public funding for many of these drugs. The future is likely to see pricing and reimbursement more closely linked with the introduction of more sophisticated 'value-based pricing' where health care providers reimburse manufacturers in a way that promotes innovation and reflects complex societal preferences for health gain.

7.6 **Conclusions**

Several approaches have been outlined including different schedules and therapeutic agents. Which approach to take depends primarily how well the patient is likely to tolerate chemotherapy and patient choice. Beyond this a more aggressive approach should be taken if the patient has potentially resectable metastatic disease (Chapters 10 and 11). Similarly if patients are symptomatic then maximizing the chance of response will heighten the chances of improving quality of life and survival. If a patient is asymptomatic then a staged combination approach can be considered or even a period of careful observation if the disease is of low volume.

The KRAS status is able to identify patients that maybe harmed by EGFR targeted therapy. In the UK the use of EGFR and VEGF targeted agents continues to be explored in randomized controlled trials. Internationally these agents have been established in routine clinical practise. Other potential predictive biomarkers have been identified in retrospective studies to guide the use of combination chemotherapy and are now being tested in a prospective randomized study.

Multiple studies have suggested a more vigilant approach as highlighted by frequent use of 2nd line chemotherapy and compliance with clinical trial protocols translates into improved survival and should therefore be encouraged.

The art of medicine is to utilize the evidence that we have and apply it to individuals to determine the most appropriate treatment.

Suggested reading

Amado RG, Wolf M, Peeters M et al. (2008) Wild-type KRAS is required for Panitumumab Efficacy in Patients with Metastatic Colorectal Cancer. *Journal of Clinical Oncology* **26**: 1626–34.

DeVita VT, Hellman S, Rosenberg SA. *Cancer Principles and Practice of Oncology*. 7th edn. www.LWWonoclogy.com.

Hurwitz H, Fehrenbacher L, Novotny W et al. (2004) Bevacizumab plus irinotecan, fluorouracil, and leucovorin for metastatic colorectal cancer. *New England Journal of Medicine* **350**: 2335–42.

Kelly C, Cassidy J (2007) Capecitabine in the treatment of colorectal cancer. *Expert Review of Anticancer Therapy* **7**: 803–10.

Malet-Martino M, Martino R (2002) Clinical studies of three oral prodrugs of 5-fluorouracil (capecitabine, UFT, S-1): A Review. *The Oncologist* **7**: 288–323.

Maughan T, Adams RA, Smith CG et al. (2009) Addition of cetuximab to oxaliplatin-based combination chemotherapy (CT) in patients with KRAS wild-type advanced colorectal cancer (ACRC): a randomised superiority trial (MRC COIN). *European Journal of Cancer Supplements* **7**: 4.

Rothenberg ML, Amit M. Oza, Robert H. Bigelow et al. (2003) Superiority of Oxaliplatin and Fluorouracil-Leucovorin Compared With Either Therapy Alone in Patients With Progressive Colorectal Cancer After Irinotecan and Fluorouracil-Leucovorin: Interim Results of a Phase III Trial. *Journal of Clinical Oncology* **21**: 2059–69.

Seymour MT, Maughan TS, Ledermann JA et al. (2007) Different strategies of sequential and combination chemotherapy for patients with poor prognosis advanced colorectal cancer (MRC FOCUS): a randomised controlled trial. *Lancet* **370**: 143–52.

Chapter 8

Surgery for recurrent rectal and colonic cancer

Peter M. Sagar

Key points

- Patients with recurrent colonic or rectal cancer need careful preoperative evaluation
- Surgical resection offers potential for cure and good palliation
- Management is multidisciplinary
- Site of recurrence determines nature of resection and prognosis.

8.1 Introduction

Surgical resection remains the principle treatment modality for rectal cancer. Although surgical techniques continue to evolve, and neo-adjuvant therapies have been adopted widely, local recurrence remains a significant problem—reported series suggest it occurs in 5–15% of patients. Affected patients face the prospect of a painful death from a malodorous, fungating recurrent tumour.

Recurrence typically occurs within the first 2 years after primary surgery, and without treatment is associated with a very poor prognosis. Median survival without treatment is about 6–7 months, and is frequently accompanied by refractory pelvic pain, uncontrollable tenesmus, and unpleasant discharge. Non operative approaches to management such as radiotherapy or chemo-radiotherapy may increase this figure to just over 12 months, albeit with the potential for disabling side-effects. Furthermore, up to two thirds of patients gain little symptomatic relief, and significant downsizing of disease is rare. Indeed, the median duration of pain relief after radiotherapy may be as little as 4 months.

About one half of patients with local recurrence of rectal cancer either have no spread outwith the pelvis or have operable hepatic or pulmonary metastases. Radical surgery for such pelvic recurrences is demanding and was previously associated with a high morbidity and mortality. Improvements in surgical technique have led to better outcomes for patients than was formerly the case. Experienced gained in the major institutions means that such patients should be carefully assessed and offered surgical intervention were appropriate.

8.2 Principles of treatment

The surgical approach to locally recurrent rectal cancer needs to be tailored for each patient and is determined by the precise location of the recurrence, invasion of adjacent organs and the proximity of major anatomical structures. Although several classification systems have been proposed in the past to aid in decision making, none are universally accepted. Table 8.1 shows a useful, practical way to subdivide the sites of local recurrence. Radical resection may be defined as resection that is achieved without the need for resection of any other pelvic organ. Extended radical resections are characterized by resections involving at least one adjacent pelvic organ, bony structure (e.g. sacrum), or major vessel (e.g. iliac vessel).

Table 8.1 Classification system for location of recurrent rectal cancer

Anatomical region	Definition
Central	Tumour confined to pelvic organs or connective tissue without contact onto or invasion into bone or pelvic side wall
Sacral	Tumour present in the presacral space with direct contact or invasion into the sacrum
Pelvic sidewall	Tumour involves the lateral pelvic sidewall with potential for invasion through the greater sciatic foramen or into piriformis and the gluteal region
Composite	Sacral and sidewall recurrence combined

8.3 Pre-operative preparations

The management of patients with recurrent rectal cancer needs to be multi-disciplinary with the combined efforts from several surgical specialists and experience in resection and/or reconstruction of abdomino-pelvic structures is essential.

Patients suitable for resection are counseled by the lead clinician with a specialist nurse, and undergo a meticulous pre-operative assessment.

Table 8.2 Contraindications to surgery for recurrent rectal cancer

Relative contraindications	Absolute contraindications
• Distant metastases • Extensive pelvic side wall involvement • Predicted R2 resection • Sacral invasion above S2-S3 junction	• Encasement of external iliac vessels • Extension of tumour through the sciatic notch • Presence of lower limb oedema from lymphatic or venous obstruction • Poor performance status

Pre-operative investigations are used to stage the disease; identify any contra-indications to surgery (Table 8.2); evaluate medical co-morbidity; and identify inoperable metastases. Staging investigations include computed tomography (CT) of the chest, abdomen and pelvis to identify metastases, magnetic resonance imaging (MRI) of the pelvis and/or liver to accurately site the recurrence or associated hepatic metastases; and 18F-flurodeoxyglucose positron emission tomography (FDG-PET) to spot occult activity.

Patients who are radiotherapy-naïve should receive long-course (5 weeks) chemo-radiotherapy, and after an interval of about 8 weeks, are re-imaged before resection. Although the disease can be downsized and down-staged by chemo-radiotherapy, the operative procedure is principally determined by the extent of the disease seen on the original scans.

Most resections are achieved via an abdominal approach although selected cases such as perineal recurrence after abdominal perineal excision may only require a perineal or posterior approach. For abdominal or composite operations, patients are placed in the modified Lloyd-Davies position, while the prone jack-knife position is employed for posterior approaches. Operative aids such as ureteric stents and tattooing of surface markings for the level of sacrectomy may be employed.

8.4 **Operative technique**

For abdominal approaches, a midline laparotomy is used to enter the abdominal cavity, and following a thorough adhesiolysis, the presence of occult intra-abdominal metastatic disease is excluded. The identification of unrecognized peritoneal metastases is a poor prognostic indicator. The aim of resection is to achieve an R0 resection. Removal of adjacent, involved organs should be en bloc. Doubt may exist about the ideal margin of excision, especially in the presence of radiotherapy induced fibrosis. Frozen section of suspect areas may help.

8.5 **Central recurrences**

Several scenarios are possible for centrally placed recurrences depending on gender, and whether the urogenital structures are involved, each demanding different operative approaches. Isolated perineal recurrences can be tackled by a trans-perineal route often with en bloc excision of the distal sacrum as this allows good exposure. When urogenital structures are involved, an *en bloc* resection is employed taking the involved viscera. While involvement of the dome of the bladder requires a partial cystectomy, involvement of the trigone demands a total cystectomy. Rarely, where the disease may involve the prostate alone (Figure 8.1) with the bladder spared, a radical prostatectomy and reconstruction, may be performed, In female patients with invasion into the vagina or uterus, a hysterectomy and either partial or complete vaginectomy is performed. Preoperative ureteric stenting helps to reduce the chance of damage to the ureters. For central recurrences that spare the urogenital structures, if the original operation was an anterior resection, the re-resection is conducted outside of the previous planes of dissection in order to avoid positive margins, and where the anastamosis is high, re-anastamosis of colon to the distal rectum may be performed. Frequently however, a non-restorative procedure such as an ultra-low Hartmann's procedure or APER is necessary. The previous anastomosis is the site of greatest weakness and excessive traction to the neo-rectum and anastomosis must be avoided during mobilization because of fear of violation of the bowel and tumour. Ideally, the plane anterior to Denonvillier's fascia is chosen for the anterior dissection. If the original operation was an APER, the small bowel falls down into the pelvis and, if involved, must be resected en bloc with the recurrent tumour mass.

The extent of the nodal dissection required in multi-visceral resections for recurrent rectal cancer is not known Invasion into other viscera opens up new lymphatic drainage systems to the disease, and ideally these should be included in the resection to limit further recurrence. However, radical pelvic lymphadenectomy adds to the morbidity.

8.6 **Sacral recurrences**

Selected posterior recurrences (Figures 8.2 and 8.3) are suitable for curative resection by an extended radical resection that includes the sacrum. The key anatomical level is at the junction of the S2/3 sacral segments. Sacral resection above this level is associated with an exceptionally high morbidity with motor and sensory neuropathies, bladder denervation, and major pelvic instability that requires reconstruction are the main limiting factors. Involvement of the sacrum

Figure 8.1 Recurrence at top of Hartmann's stump with anterior invasion into the prostate

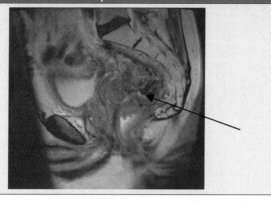

with recurrent tumour below this level is optimally managed with a distal sacrectomy with en bloc resection of the neo-rectum or mass. Occasionally, the anterior cortex of S1 or S2 is involved, and the surgeon may consider excision of the tumour mass combined with the bony cortex of the affected segments. Where the fascia over the sacrum or the periosteum are involved but the bone is clear of the tumour, a trial dissection may show that the fascia can be lifted off with the tumour mass leaving the bony sacrum intact. Sacral resection is usually conducted via a two-stage composite abdomino-sacral approach. For the first stage, the patient is placed in the Lloyd-Davies position and the abdomen is entered through a midline laparotomy. After a comprehensive adhesiolysis, the ureters and iliac vessels are identified and isolated. Where there is a significant lateral pelvic sidewall component of disease recurrence, the internal iliac vessels may be ligated, typically aiming to preserve the first branch of the vessel in order to promote skin and muscle flap healing. The tumour mass with any associated neo-rectum or rectal stump is then mobilized anteriorly, laterally, and where possible inferiorly with careful attention to avoid violating the tumour. Any attached viscera are resected en bloc. Once the tumour mass is attached posteriorly only, stomas and ileal conduits are constructed, drains placed, and where possible an omentoplasty used to fill the pelvis prior to closure of the abdomen. The patient is then positioned in the prone jack-knife position. This has the advantage of permitting a wide *en bloc* resection with good exposure.

A vertical incision is made over the sacrum extending from the level of S1 to the perineal scar or anus. The incision is continued to the bony sacrum and the gluteal muscles are reflected laterally. The sacro-tuberous and sacro-spinous ligaments are divided laterally to

Figure 8.2 Recurrent rectal cancer lying behind the uterus and adherent but not invading the sacrum

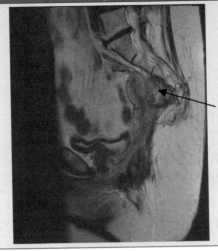

enable entry into the pelvic cavity, and access gained to the pelvic cavity. The level of sacral division is confirmed. A sacral osteotomy is made and the filiform terminale are ligated. Any residual fascial or ligamentous attachments are dissected by electro-cautery before completion of the sacrectomy and removal of the specimen *en bloc*. A combination of omentum, absorbable mesh, or pedicled flaps may be used to close the defect.

8.7 **Lateral recurrences**

Recurrence of rectal cancer that invades into the pelvic sidewall is associated with the worst prognosis and the least chance of an R0 resection. The disease often involves key structures such as the ureters, iliac vessels (with the veins particularly troublesome), or the bony pelvis itself. Extensive involvement of the pelvic sidewall is a contra-indication to surgery. The surgical approach involves pre-operative stenting of ureters to aid in their identification and estimation of involvement with disease. At operation, early control of the key structures proximal and distal to the tumour involved field is essential. Resection of the tumour and attached structures is subsequently carried out *en bloc* with reconstruction of essential vessels and re-implantation or re-routing of the ureter.

The dissection begins at the level of the pelvic brim with identification and looping of the ureters and common iliac vessels. The course of the ureter is then traced to the bladder, and further dissection

Figure 8.3 Recurrent rectal cancer invading into the lower sacrum

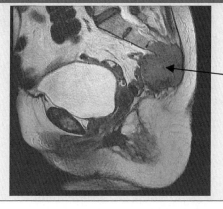

to identify and control the internal and external iliac vessels is conducted. Ligation and division of the internal iliac artery allows access to the underlying internal iliac vein, which can be similarly dealt with if inseparable from the tumour. This vessel may be taken bilaterally if necessary to achieve an R0 resection. Where practical, the internal iliac artery is ligated distal to its first branch. The first branch of the internal iliac artery subsequently divides to form the ilio-lumbar, superior gluteal, and lateral sacral arteries, and its preservation is helpful to reduce perineal or posterior wound related complications. Once the internal iliac vessels have been controlled and divided, a radical wide resection of the recurrent disease is carried out. Encouraging results have been described when the extensive lateral sidewall disease is tackled with dissection in the plane between the boney pelvis and the sidewall musculature. Using this approach an overall survival of 69% at a mean follow up of 19 months was achieved.

8.8 Results

Table 8.3 shows published results from a number of the major centres that routinely carry out resection for locally recurrent rectal cancer. Inevitably, such series are case series of a heterogenous population of patients. Morbidity and mortality, percentage of patients in whom an R0 (no microscopic disease at resection margins) as well as long term outcome will vary depending on the case mix of the particular unit and how aggressive the team is with their approach. As a rule of thumb, one third of patients are alive at five years, one third will develop metastatic disease and one third will develop further local recurrence (with some being suitable for re-resection).

Table 8.3 Outcomes from surgical series of resection for recurrent rectal cancer

Reference	Year	Study type	Centre	Number	R0 (%)	Survival measure	Morbidity (%)	Mortality (%)
Hahnloser	2003	Case series	Mayo clinic (US)	304	45	25% 5 year survival	26	<1
Moriya	2004	Case series	Tokyo (JPN)	57	84	42% 5 year survival	58	3
Boyle	2005	Case series	Leeds (UK)	64	37	Median survival 34 months	35	2
Wiig	2006	Case series	Oslo (NOR)	150	44	27% 5 year survival	46	<1
Maetani	2007	Case series	Kyoto (JPN)	61	–	19% 10 year survival	–	3
Heriot	2008	Case series	Multicentre	160	61	Median survival 43 months	27	<1
Schurr	2008	Case series	Hamburg (GER)	72	51	Median survival 55 months	15	9
Kusters	2009	Case series	Eindhoven (HOL)	170	54	40% 5 year survival	–	7

8.9 **Management of locally recurrent colonic cancer**

The principles of management of locally recurrent colonic cancer are similar to those that appertain to the management of recurrent rectal cancer within the pelvis:

- Assessment of the patient's fitness for operation
- Identification of metastatic disease
- Accurate radiological assessment of the involvement of surrounding structures.

Radiotherapy is rarely used in this setting and chemotherapy will rarely change the operability or otherwise of a tumour. Adherence to basic surgical principles of gentle handling of tissues, no-touch technique, early control of blood vessels and radical *en bloc* resection offers the chance of long term survival with good quality of life.

8.10 **Conclusions**

Recurrent rectal cancer presents a major surgical challenge but without surgery affected patients can expect an exceptionally poor quality of life with little or no hope of cure. Surgery for local recurrence now has an established place in selected patients and offers the only realistic chance of long-term survival and cure. Surgery in this setting also provides acceptable palliation in patients. Decisions about the optimal management for these patients require a multidisciplinary approach.

The published literature from major centres illustrates the value of aggressive multi-visceral resection. While not all patients with locally recurrent rectal cancer meet the criteria for resection, it is likely that, as surgical experience grows and improved chemotherapeutic regimens and preoperative radiotherapy strategies come available; more patients with recurrent disease will be cured.

Suggested reading

Bakx R, Visser O, Josso J, Meifer S, Frederik J, Slors M, van Lanschot JJB (2008) Management of recurrent rectal cancer: A population based study in greater Amsterdam. *World J Gastroenterol* **21**(14): 6018–23.

Boyle KM, Sagar PM, Chalmers AG, Sebag-Montefiore D, Cairns A, Eardley I (2005) Surgery for locally recurrent rectal cancer. *Dis Colon rectum* **48**: 929–37.

Hahnloser D, Nelson H, Gunderson LL, Hassan I, Haddock MG, O'Connell MJ, Cha S, Sargent DJ, Horgan A (2003) Curative potential of multimodality therapy for locally recurrent rectal cancer. *Ann Surg* **237**: 502–8.

Heriot AG, Byrne CM, Lee P, Dobbs B, Tilney H, Solomon MJ, Mackay J, Frizelle F (2008) Extended radical resection: the choice for locally recurrent rectal cancer. *Dis Colon Rectum* **51**: 284–91.

Moore HG, Shoup M, Riedel E, Minsky BD, Alektiar KM, Ercolani M, Paty PB, Wong WD, Guillem JG (2004) Colorectal cancer pelvic recurrences: determinants of resectability. *Dis Colon Rectum* **47**: 1599–1606.

Rao AR, Kagan AR, Chan PM, Gilbert HA, Nussbaum H, Hintz BL (1981) Patterns of recurrence following curative resection alone for adenocarcinoma of the rectum and sigmoid colon. *Cancer* **48**: 1492–5.

Sebag-Montefiore D, Stephens RJ, Steele R, Monson J, Grieve R, Khanna S, Quirke P, Couture J, de Metz C, Myint AS, Bessell E, Griffiths G, Thompson LC, Parmar M (2009) Preoperative radiotherapy versus selective postoperative chemoradiotherapy in patients with rectal cancer (MRC CR07 and NCIC CTG C016): a multicentre, randomised trial. *Lancet* **373**: 811–20.

Chapter 9

Surgery for liver metastases

Robert A. Adair, Alastair L. Young, and
Giles J. Toogood

Key points

- Up to 20% of patients present with synchronous
  liver metastases and a further 40% will develop
  metachronous liver disease
- 5 year survival following hepatic resection now
  approaches 40%
- Extra-hepatic disease is no longer considered an
  absolute contraindication to curative resection
- Management is dependent upon a multidisciplinary
  team approach in specialist, high volume, centres.

9.1 Patient selection

Until the mid-1960s elective liver resection carried a mortality
rate of 15% or higher. Technical improvements around this time
occurred mainly as a result of military surgery and a more detailed
understanding of internal liver anatomy. Couinaud first described
the now conventional, segmental anatomy of the liver in the 1950s
(Figure 9.1). This newly acquired knowledge coupled with the open-
ing of a school of liver surgery in Paris in the 1960s by Bismuth, led to
significant improvements in surgical techniques. With the development of specialized Hepatobiliary units, mortality rates for elective
liver resection are now below 5%.

Whilst improvements in surgical techniques have contributed
to better outcomes, other factors have also played an important
role. Improvements in cross sectional and magnetic resonance
imaging have enabled optimal surgical planning prior to resection.
The use of intra-operative ultrasound scanning enables precise
tumour localization. Modern anaesthetic techniques such as low

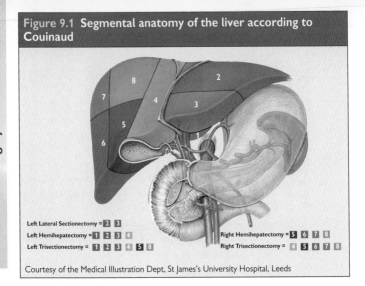

Figure 9.1 Segmental anatomy of the liver according to Couinaud

Left Lateral Sectionectomy = 2 3
Left Hemihepatectomy = 1 2 3 4
Left Trisectionectomy = 1 2 3 4 5 8

Right Hemihepatectomy = 5 6 7 8
Right Trisectionectomy = 4 5 6 7 8

Courtesy of the Medical Illustration Dept, St James's University Hospital, Leeds

central venous pressure anaesthesia have significantly reduced intra-operative blood loss without detriment to renal or hepatic perfusion. Modern critical care facilities have enhanced postoperative care but perhaps the most important development is the multidisciplinary approach with care individualized to each patient.

Historically, liver resection was restricted to those without extra-hepatic disease who had four or less unilobar tumours measuring no more than 5 cm in diameter. Much of this dogma centred around the characteristics of the primary tumour. Several clinical risk scores have been developed based on tumour related factors. Using regression analysis, Fong et al. found five tumour related characteristics in 1,001 patients which predicted prognosis. These included node-positive primary disease, carcinoembryonic antigen (CEA) greater than 200 ng/mL, greater than one liver lesion, any lesion greater than 5 cm, and disease free interval less than one year from resection of the primary lesion. Rees et al .found similar characteristics predicted outcome in their study of 929 patients.

Extensive work focusing on the liver remaining following resection—the future liver remnant (FLR) has resulted in a paradigm shift in defining resectability of colorectal liver metastasis (CRLM). In 2006 the American Hepato-Pancreato-Biliary Association (AHPBA), Society of Surgical Oncology (SSO), and Society for Surgery of Alimentary Tract (SSAT) issued a consensus statement which focused on the ability to obtain margin-negative resection (R0) while leaving a FLR consisting of at least two contiguous hepatic sectors, adequate inflow, outflow, biliary drainage, and a greater than 20% FLR of liver volume in a healthy liver. As such very few tumour related factors are now taken as a contraindication to resection (Table 9.1).

Table 9.1 **Types of major liver resections**	
Name	**Segments Resected**
Right Hemihepatectomy	5,6,7,8
Right Trisectionectomy	4,5,6,7,8 (+/− 1)
Left Hemihepatectomy	2,3,4
Left Trisectionectomy	2,3,4,5,8 (+/− 1)

A FLR of 20% is now generally accepted as a definition of resectability for CRLM meaning that up to 80% of the liver can be resected if necessary provided the underlying parenchyma is normal. The estimation of required FLR is not only volumetric. Function after resection must be estimated as a correlation between FLR and postoperative outcome has been established. Most centres use a combination of computed tomography (CT) and magnetic resonance imaging (MRI). FLR can be measured directly by CT and is standardized to the patient's size using a formula which relates liver volume to body surface area. Larger FLRs must be maintained in the presence of diseased parenchyma. It is generally accepted that a FLR of up to 30% and 40% must remain for mild and severe parenchymal disease respectively.

The removal of all macroscopic tumour with negative resection margins remains the gold standard of the surgical treatment of CRLM. However the importance of margin negative (R0) resection has been the focus of debate in recent years. Positive resection margins have historically been associated with reduced overall survival. It was widely held that a clear resection margin measuring 1 cm was required. Pawlik's study demonstrated however, that resection margins of at least one centimetre did not demonstrate a statistically significant difference in recurrence rate, site of recurrence, or overall survival compared with those patients who had a close (1–4 mm) margin. This prompted the SSO consensus statement of 2006 that whilst wide margins should be sought, the anticipation of close margins should not preclude resection. In 2008 de Hass et al. reported that overall survival in 234 R1 resections approached that of the 202 in the R0 group. This is likely to be due to improvements in cytotoxic therapy and supports the use of aggressive surgical resection even when a negative resection margin is not attainable in selected patients.

9.2 **Techniques**

Resections for CRLM can be classified as anatomical or non-anatomical, major or minor. Anatomical resection involves removal of a Couninaud segment or segments whilst non anatomical resection involves the removal of the tumour itself with a margin of normal liver tissue. Major resection is defined as the removal of three or more Couninaud segments.

9.2.1 **Synchronous disease**

The management of patients presenting with synchronous disease presents an interesting challenge. Two approaches can be adopted. A staged approach where the primary disease is resected first followed by liver resection. In some cases concomitant resection of both may be undertaken at one operation. Several studies have been conducted comparing the two approaches as concerns had been raised about the safety of synchronous resection. Theoretical tumour seeding in the FLR caused concerns as did the perceived increase risk of infection associated with colonic surgery.

In a study of 610 patients by Reddy et al., major hepatectomy in synchronous resection was associated with poorer outcome whereas simultaneous minor resection was safe with shorter hospital stay. In a more recent study however, Martin et al. reported comparable outcomes in 70 patients undergoing simultaneous major hepatic resection when compared with 160 undergoing a staged procedure. They concluded that simultaneous resection was safe and that cumulative hospital stay was reduced in the simultaneous group.

Historically, factors such as primary tumour bleeding, perforation or the development of intestinal obstruction have been used to support a primary first approach in the management of synchronous disease. More recently however, small studies have examined the role of liver first surgery. Patients were treated with chemotherapy prior to liver resection with surgery for their asymptomatic primary tumour deferred. No differences were reported in median survival or peri-operative outcomes. The practice of liver directed surgery first is not one which is widely accepted however, perhaps due to patient selection based on prognostic factors associated with the primary tumour historically.

9.2.2 **Portal Vein Embolisation**

PVE was first described as a method of increasing the size of the FLR in 1990. Utilised in those with increased risk of hepatic insufficiency after resection, PVE enables hypertrophy of the FLR prior to resection—in essence hepatic regeneration has begun prior to resection. Patients where this may prove beneficial include those with background cirrhosis or chemotherapy induced steatohepatitis. The prinicple is ligation or embolization of the portal vein supplying all tumour-bearing liver allowing hypertrophy of the contralateral FLR. Employing this technique can render operable and therefore potentially cure an increasing cohort of patients with sub-optimal FLRs.

9.2.3 **Two Stage Hepatectomy**

Patients with bilobar multifocal disease pose a challenge. Traditionally considered inoperable, improvements in cytotoxic regimens have meant that for many, two stage resection can be a viable option. Often chemotherapy is utilized in an attempt to downstage tumour burden and may give some indication as to the tumour biology. Progression of bilobar, multifocal disease despite chemotherapy precludes an aggressive surgical approach. Chemotherapy is not without consequence. Steatohepatitis and sinusoidal obstructive syndrome (SOS) associated with irinotecan and oxaliplatin based regimes can compromise the FLR making extended resection in borderline patients even more challenging. CT assessment of spleen size or resovist MRI may predict the presence of SOS ahead of surgery.

The choice of which side to address 1st depends on the distribution of the disease. The preponderance for CRLM to affect the right lobe of the liver is thought to be due to flow dynamics in the portal system and in part its size. Hence most surgeons advocate a right side first approach. This permits the left FLR to hypertrophy and allow a second left sided resection. What is apparent from the current literature is that careful surgical planning, estimation of the FLR, and patient selection are of paramount importance. Completion rates range from 76–100% with favourable overall survival.

9.2.4 **Radiological complete response**

Complete response rates following chemotherapy are <5% for single agent fluoropyrimidines (Fu) and <10% for combination chemotherapy even when triplet agent chemotherapy is used. Post resection viable tumour cells are seen in over 80% contain of resection specimens. The surgical strategy should therefore be to remove all known tumours.

9.2.5 **Extrahepatic disease**

Historically extrahepatic disease was associated with poor outcome and precluded surgery due to reports of poor survival. The combination of modern systemic therapy and an aggressve surgical approach has yielded 5 year overall survival rates reaching 45%. Patients with portal lymphadenopathy or peritoneal disease however should still be managed non-surgically.

9.2.6 **Ablataive techniques**

Ablative therapies have been developed utilizing cooling, cryoablation or heat, radio frequency ablation (RFA). The latter is used more commonly and aims to destroy the tumour with a rim of normal parenchyma. A probe is placed in the tumour percutaneously, during an open procedure or laparoscopically. It is used mainly in patients where the preservation of parenchyma is important.

Many studies have attempted to directly compare RFA with resection. Recurrence rates vary in these studies from around 2% to over 80%. Increasing tumour size to greater than 3 cm has been shown to be associated with higher rates of recurrence. A loss of heat to surrounding blood vessels during ablation may produce a heat sink effect, lowering the temperature leading to suboptimal necrosis. Percutaneous approaches have also been shown to have higher recurrence rates.

New generation microwave and Nd-Yag ablation techniques may reduce the impact of the heat sink effect but prospective randomized studies are required to assess their overall benefit.

9.3 **Outcomes**

Outcomes for stage IV colorectal cancer have improved dramatically over the past decade. Whilst no randomised data is available to support the role of metastectomy compelling survival data from multiple case series has convinced the international oncology community of its worth. A recent randomized trial (EPOC) of perioperative chemotherapy plus surgery versus surgery failed to show a significant benefit for the experimental arm on intent to treat analysis. However this provided 30% 5 year survival data in a controlled setting following metastectomy.

The low rates of perioperative mortality and short length inpatient of stays now achieved in specialist centres make surgery an attractive option. However the magnitude of difference it makes can only truly be determined by a randomised clinical trial. A feasibility study, Pulmonary Metastasectomy in Colorectal Cancer (PulMiCC) to assess whether such a study could be successfully conducted is currently underway in the UK (see Chapter 10).

Suggested reading

Charnsangavej C, Clary B, Fong Y, et al. (2006) Selection of patients for resection of hepatic colorectal metastases: expert consensus statement. *Ann Surg Oncol* **13**(10): 1261–8.

de Haas RJ, Wicherts DA, Flores E, et al. (2008) R1 resection by necessity for colorectal liver metastases: is it still a contraindication to surgery? *Ann Surg* **248**(4): 626–37.

Fong Y, Fortner J, Sun RL, et al. (1999) Clinical Score for Predicting Recurrence After Hepatic Resection for Metastatic Colorectal CancerAnalysis of 1001 Consecutive Cases. *Ann Surg* **230**(3): 309–18; discussion 318–21.

Martin RC 2nd, Augenstein V, Reuter NP, Scoggins CR, McMasters KM (2009) Simultaneous versus staged resection for synchronous colorectal cancer liver metastases. *J Am Coll Surg* **208**: 842–50, discussion 850–2.

Pawlik TM, Scoggins CR, Zorzi D, et al. (2005) Effect of surgical margin status on survival and site of recurrence after hepatic resection for colorectal metastases. *Ann Surg* **241**(5): 715–22.

Reddy SK, Pawlik TM, Zorzi D, Gleisner AL, Ribero D, Assumpcao L, Barbas AS, Abdalla EK, Choti MA, Vauthey JN, et al. (2007) Simultaneous resections of colorectal cancer and synchronous liver metastases: a multi-institutional analysis. *Annals of Surgical Oncology* **14**: 3481–91.

Rees M, Tekkis PP, Welsh FK, O'Rourke T, John TG (2008) Evaluation of long-term survival after hepatic resection for metastatic colorectal cancer: a multifactorial model of 929 patients. *Ann Surg* **247**(1): 125–35.

Chapter 10

Surgery for pulmonary metastases

Ian S. Morgan and David R. Ferry

> **Key points**
> - Pulmonary metastasectomy for colorectal cancer is practiced widely but evidence for its effectiveness is lacking
> - A multidisciplinary team approach is recommended to select cases who may benefit from intervention
> - Patients who fall within the zone of uncertainty should be entered into a clinical trial
> - Surgical management should aim to remove all metastatic disease whilst preserving lung parenchyma
> - Five year survival following metastasectomy is over 40% in selected cases.

10.1 Patient selection

Colorectal cancer forms the largest group for pulmonary metastasectomy and is becoming increasingly accepted as standard practice. However, a web-based survey of European surgeons has revealed wide variations in selection and technique of pulmonary metastasectomy for colorectal cancer (PMCC). Evidence for PMCC is weak, but usually justified by extrapolation of data from hepatic metastasectomy.

The following general principles should be considered in assessing the suitability of a patient for PMCC (Box 10.1).

The primary colon tumour should have been resected with the intention of cure. In cases where radical resection is considered, then pulmonary metastasectomy may be performed initially.

Resectable extrathoracic metastases do not contra-indicate PMCC, particularly with hepatic metastases.

> ### Box 10.1 General principles
>
> **Disease factors**
>
> • Control of primary tumour
> • No extrathoracic metastatic disease except hepatic metastases suitable for resection
> • Complete resection of all metastatic disease anticipated.
>
> **Patient factors**
>
> • Patient is operable—i.e. able to withstand surgery at an acceptable risk, and tolerate the extent of planned resection.

Complete resection of all metastases must be feasible, whilst preserving adequate lung parenchyma. Incomplete resections confer no benefit.

10.2 Patient evaluation

The majority of pulmonary metastases are detected coincidentally in asymptomatic patients by plain chest radiology or during surveillance CT scan. Solitary pulmonary lesions should be evaluated as possible lung cancer even in the presence of hepatic metastases. This may require CT-guided biopsy or surgical resection after excluding metastatic disease. Positron emission tomography (PET) scanning is a valuable adjunct in excluding extrathoracic metastatic disease and mediastinal nodal disease, but is limited by a minimum size resolutuion of 5 to 8 mm. Up to 15% of pulmonary metastases have associated involvement of mediastinal nodes, so consideration should be given to assessing the mediastinum by mediastinoscopy or other modalities (endobronchial ultrasound [EBUS], endoscopic ultrasound [EUS]).

The patient should have sufficient fitness to tolerate the surgical procedure in terms of comorbidities, such as cardiac and renal disease. These should be evaluated as per current British Thoracic Society guidelines. Finally the extent of resection should not result in respiratory compromise, as assessed by preoperative lung function.

10.3 Systemic therapy

The role of adjuvant chemotherapy after resection of the primary colon cancer is discussed in Chapter 6. The value of chemotherapy or radiotherapy following PMCC is not well established. Where patients are chemotherapy naïve adjuvant therapy is commonly considered.

10.4 Techniques

The relative merits of open versus minimally invasive surgery have not yet been resolved. Despite the accuracy of current CT scanners in identifying small pulmonary lesions, the detection of further unsuspected lesions at thoracotomy remains high.

10.4.1 Surgical approaches

- **Thoracotomy** involves a major incision through the chest wall requiring division of large muscles and enlarging the intercostal space with a retractor to gain access to the thoracic cavity. This facilitates bimanual palpation of lung parenchyma and evaluation of hilar and mediastinal lymph nodes
- **Posterolateral thoracotomy** through the fifth interspace is a popular approach for PMCC. The latissimus dorsi muscle is usually divided, although serratus anterior is often preserved. Nevertheless, this major incision results in significant morbidity with prolonged recovery
- **Muscle-sparing** incisions limit pain and functional impairment allowing early recovery
- **Axillary thoracotomy and minithoracotomy (lateral or anterior)** are alternatives to the muscle-sparing approach
- **Median sternotomy** is utilized for bilateral metastases and is well tolerated in terms of functional recovery although access to the left lower lobe is more challenging. An alternative bilateral staged approach should be considered and is the preferred approach for the majority of surgeons. For a planned two-stage approach, the side with the larger or greater number of metastases is operated first, followed by the contralateral side 3 to 6 weeks later
- **Bilateral anterior thoracotomy or clamshell incision** provides good access to both lower lobes and is an alternative to median sternotomy
- **Video-assisted thoracoscopic surgery (VATS)** has gained in popularity during the last two decades, with major lung resections feasible and now performed routinely. Shorter hospital stays and more rapid functional recovery make this an attractive option. However, the lack of bimanual palpation to detect occult pulmonary metastases may limit the usefulness of minimally invasive approaches in this setting.

10.4.2 Resection techniques

The technique applied to resection of PMCC is largely dictated by the approach. Thoracotomy, despite being an invasive incision, allows for more precise and limited resection thus preserving lung parenchyma. VATS generally requires the use of surgical staplers which resects a larger margin of lung, but with a more rapid recovery from surgery.

- **Precision excision—diathermy or laser** is used to resect peripheral and deeper lesions with minimal sacrifice of normal lung parenchyma. At least partial inflation of the lung is required, so this method is usually performed via thoracotomy or other open approaches
- **Stapled wedge resection (Figure 10.1)** is ideally suited to VATS resection of peripheral lesions. A wider margin of lung parenchyma is removed, limiting its usefulness in multiple lesions or patients with poor lung reserve.

Figure 10.1 **A) CT scan of peripheral lesion in right upper lobe B) VATS** stapled wedge resection of right upper lobe lesion

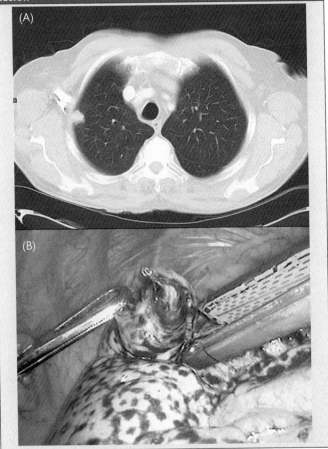

- **Anatomic segmentectomy, lobectomy or pneumonectomy** results in a much greater loss of lung tissue, with associated physiologic consequences and significantly higher mortality and morbidity. A careful assessment is necessary before undertaking such major resections, but may be justified in highly selected cases

- **Image-Guided Ablative techniques** (thermoablative therapies) are novel less-invasive methods. The techniques currently available are: radiofrequency ablation, microwave ablation and cryoablation. Their use is discussed in relation to hepatic metastases in Chapter 9

- **Mediastinal lymph node** involvement is reported in 10–15% of cases presenting with colorectal pulmonary metastases, and is associated with much poorer survival. Since the primary aim of metastasectomy is removal of all disease, this cannot be achieved when mediastinal nodes are involved. Accurate assessment of mediastinal nodes therefore is essential, and is generally best established by mediastinoscopy

- **Concurrent hepatic metastases** with pulmonary metastases deserve special consideration. The timing and order of surgery should be discussed jointly between thoracic and hepatobiliary surgical teams. Solitary pulmonary lesions should probably be resected first, on the basis that a proportion of these will be primary lung cancer which is biologically more aggressive. Otherwise, initial hepatic resection, particularly if there is doubt regarding resectability, would seem logical.

10.5 **Outcomes**

Perioperative mortality following pulmonary resection is currently 0–2%, depending on comorbidities, and extent of resection. Five year survival results are variable and are influenced by a number of prognostic factors. For the most favourable cases, at least 40% 5 year survival has been reported.

10.5.1 **Prognostic factors (Box 10.2)**

Disease free interval of greater than 1 year prior to detection of pulmonary metastases is associated with improved survival. Usually patients are selected for PMCC with limited number of metastases, with over 50% solitary. Greater numbers of metastases are associated with poorer survival. However, unlike primary lung cancer, tumour size does not appear to be a factor. The majority of series report mediastinal lymph node involvement as an ominous prognostic factor. Concurrent hepatic and pulmonary metastases have not been demonstrated to adversely affect outcome, although large

- Disease free interval
- Number of metastases
- Mediastinal lymph node involvement
- Hepatic metastases
- CEA.

Abbreviations: CEA: Serum carcinoembryonic antigen level

liver metastases (>3 cm) at the time of primary tumour resection is a poor prognostic indicator. Levels of CEA are poorly reported in studies, but elevated levels do appear to be associated with poorer survival.

Follow-up and surveillance should continue after PMCC with CT scans at 6 monthly intervals for 2 years, then yearly. Repeat PMCC should be considered in cases of recurrence and is associated with a low mortality and good 5 year survival.

10.6 **PulMiCC trial**

In order to address shortcomings in the evidence base for pulmonary metastasectomy, a randomized trial called pulmonary metastasectomy in colorectal cancer (PulMiCC) opened to recruitment to 14 UK centres in March 2010. This feasibility study will establish if sufficient patients can be recruited prior to conducting a larger randomized trial. Secondary endpoints are: overall survival, relapse-free survival, lung function, self-reported quality of life and health economic assessment. The study design is outlined in Figure 10.2.

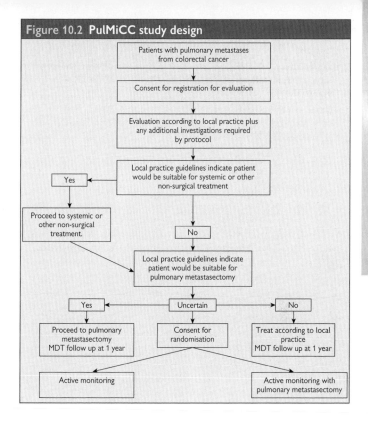

Figure 10.2 PulMiCC study design

Patients with pulmonary metastases from colorectal cancer

↓

Consent for registration for evaluation

↓

Evaluation according to local practice plus any additional investigations required by protocol

↓

Local practice guidelines indicate patient would be suitable for systemic or other non-surgical treatment

Yes → Proceed to systemic or other non-surgical treatment.

No ↓

Local practice guidelines indicate patient would be suitable for pulmonary metastasectomy

Yes → Proceed to pulmonary metastasectomy MDT follow up at 1 year

Uncertain → Consent for randomisation

No → Treat according to local practice MDT follow up at 1 year

Active monitoring

Active monitoring with pulmonary metastasectomy

Suggested reading

Fiorentino F, Hunt I, Teoh K, et al. (2010) Pulmonary metastasectomy in colorectal cancer: a systematic review and quantitative synthesis. *J R Soc Med* **103**: 60–6.

Internullo E, Cassivi SD, Van Raemdonck D, Friedel G, Treasure T (2008) Pulmonary metastasectomy: a survey of current practice amongst members of the European Society of Thoracic Surgeons. *J Thorac Oncol* **3**(11): 1257–66.

Lee WS, Yun SH, Chun HK, et al. (2006) Pulmonary resection for metastases from colorectal cancer: prognostic factors and survival. *Int J Colorectal Dis* **22**(6): 699–704.

Lin BR, Chang TC, Lee YC, et al. (2009) Pulmonary resection for colorectal cancer metastases: duration between cancer onset and lung metastasis as an important prognostic factor. *Ann Surg Oncol* **16**: 102632.

Pfannschmidt J, Dienemann H, Hoffmann H (2007) Surgical resection of pulmonary metastases from colorectal cancer: a systematic review of published series. *Ann Thorac Surg* **84**(1): 324–38.

Pfannschmidt J, Hoffmann H, Dienemann H (2010) Factors influencing outcome of pulmonary metastasectomy for colorectal cancer. *J Thorac Oncol.* **5**: S172–8.

Welter S, Jacobs J, Krbek T, et al. (2007) Long-term survival after repeated resection of pulmonary metastases from colorectal cancer. *Ann Thorac Surg* **84**: 203–10.

Welter S, Jacobs J, Krbek T, et al. (2007) Prognostic impact of lymph node involvement in pulmonary metastases from colorectal cancer. *Eur J Cardiothorac Surg* **31**: 1672.

Chapter 11

Colorectal cancer–surgical and non-surgical palliation

Christopher Macklin and Bill Hulme

> **Key points**
> - Approximately half of patients with colorectal will die of their disease and a significant proportion will need surgical and/or medical palliation
> - Decision making involving the patient and the palliative care and surgical teams is paramount to ensure appropriate and timely treatment
> - Malignant bowel obstruction can be relieved through a variety of surgical interventions or ameliorated pharmacologically
> - Tenesmus or unacceptable rectal symptoms may need a combined approach for symptom control.

11.1 Background

Colorectal cancer is common with a 4% lifetime incidence and although surgery is the primary treatment, cure is achieved in only approximately 50% of patients. From a surgical point of view, therapy may be considered palliative when the resection of all known cancer is no longer possible. The remit of the surgeon has expanded in recent times and radical approaches are now considered in selected patients with local recurrence and metastatic disease with 5 year survival rates approximating to 30% (see Chapters 8, 9, and 10).

Decisions regarding whether to pursue a surgical or conservative approach need to be made with the full consultation of the patient and their next of kin. There are a number of difficult concepts with competing interests such as the risks of surgical mortality and morbidity, recovery time versus benefits in terms of quality and quantity of life, and patient preference. Often, these discussions fall to the surgeon closely involved with the case with support from the MDT particularly the colorectal nurse specialists, palliative care team and oncologists. Adequate training should be provided to ensure high quality and empathic consultations.

11.2 Malignant bowel obstruction

11.2.1 Surgical approach

Once the decision has been made that the patient is fit for a procedure then there needs to be consideration as to the risk/benefit of particular interventions. Options available are endoluminal stenting, laser recanalisation, laparoscopic or open surgery with an aim to resect, bypass or defunction the obstruction by means of a stoma.

11.2.1.1 Endoluminal stenting

Colorectal stenting has been performed since the early 1990s and the gold standard in modern times is the self-expanding metal stent often placed as a combined endoscopic radiological procedure. Success rates are commonly in excess of 80% (decreasing with more proximal lesions and around the flexures) and complications include perforation, migration, bleeding, tenesmus (in mid and low rectal tumours) and tumour ingrowth with re-obstruction.

11.2.1.2 Laser recanalization

Laser recanalization is less useful for complete obstruction than stenting but is particularly good in partially obstructing rectal cancers where bleeding and tenesmus also feature and stenting would worsen tenesmus. Laser may also be used in conjunction with stenting to treat regrowth.

11.2.1.3 Laparoscopic and open surgery

The laparoscopic approach has been found to result in quicker recovery which is of paramount importance to patients with limited life expectancy. Laparoscopic surgery is not always possible especially in patients with multiple previous procedures and/or carcinomatosis peritonei but should be considered for surgical palliation when the appropriate equipment and skills are available.

Mortality from surgery for palliation of colorectal cancer can be as high as 25% or more. Although some studies have demonstrated a survival advantage for patients fit for resection there is no randomized data to support resection and decisions should be made on a case by case basis. Some indicators that worsen survival are low albumin, high CEA, more than 25% liver replacement with metastases, more than 100 mls of ascitic fluid and multiple metastatic sites of disease.

Irresectable disease can be treated by bypass to try and avoid a stoma at the risk of an anastomosis but in many cases a defunctioning stoma can be the quickest, easiest and lowest morbidity procedure.

11.2.1.4 Deciding which patients are unsuitable for surgery

As outlined above, reaching a decision on whether a patient would benefit from palliative surgery for malignant bowel obstruction is complex and often involves wide discussion. There are a number of patients who are more likely to benefit from surgery and essentially they are those who:

1. Are willing to undergo surgery
2. Have an obstruction due to a discrete mechanical lesion
3. Have a good performance status
4. Have not had relief of symptoms following 48–72 hours of conservative medical management.

Conversely patients who are unlikely to benefit from surgery are those:

a) With diffuse peritoneal carcinomatosis
b) With recurrent ascites
c) With distant metastases
d) Who have had previous explorative laparotomies, and where there is no likely means of reversing the obstruction.

Patients where it is thought surgery is not appropriate should still receive careful attention, with non-surgical management outlined below.

11.2.2 **Palliative approach**

For those patients with an inoperable bowel obstruction pharmaco-logical options can be effective in relieving 70–90% of associated symptoms, usually without the need for a nasogastric tube (Baines et al.). Whilst the primary approach is relief of symptoms, a proportion of patients can experience a reversal of their obstruction through conservative management, although a recurrence is likely. This approach uses analgesics for the constant pain associated with obstruction, antispasmodic agents for those patients with colic and antiemetics for nausea and vomiting. Antisecretory agents can also reduce the accumulation of intestinal fluid and therefore lessen vomiting.

Oral absorption of drugs should not be relied upon in bowel obstruction so the parenteral route is usually used, either intravenously or subcutaneously. Continuous subcutaneous infusion is often preferred by ambulant patients as analgesics and antiemetics can be combined in a single syringe and placed in a relatively small infusion device. Occasionally for patients with stable symptoms transdermal opiates and antisecretory agents can be used if parenteral routes of administration are not possible. Rectal opiates and antiemetics are also available.

11.2.2.1 Analgesics

Despite their constipating side effects opiates remain the analgesic of choice in bowel obstruction. Opiates commonly used include morphine, diamorphine, oxycodone, fentanyl, and hydromorphone. Choice is usually dictated by local availability, compatibility with other drugs in combined infusions or by other complicating medical conditions such as renal impairment, rather than one opiate being more effective than another.

By using continuous parenteral infusions careful dose titration can be achieved whilst guaranteeing effective drug delivery. Transdermal opiate patches (such as fentanyl or buprenorphine) can be used for those patients with stable pain, but dose adjustments need 12–24 hours to take effect.

11.2.2.2 Antiemetics

For those with an incomplete bowel obstruction due to a failure of peristalsis a trial of metoclopramide is used first line. As well as acting centrally this prokinetic agent increases peristaltic activity and may relieve the obstruction if there is an underlying functional cause. This approach should not be used if the patient has a complete obstruction as the resultant colicky (spasmodic) abdominal pain will be made worse, with the theoretical risk of perforation. Consideration should also be given to stopping other agents that cause colic such as stimulant laxatives, where switching to a stool softener is preferred.

For complete bowel obstruction haloperidol acts centrally to reduce nausea, and is less sedating than other antipsychotics such as prochlorperazine and levomepromazine. Dose can be titrated against effect (for usual dose ranges see Table 11.1). Alternatively cyclizine acts on both histamine and cholinergic receptors and can relieve nausea and vomiting by these mechanisms. Should either haloperidol or cyclizine fail individually to relieve symptoms they can be used simultaneously or replaced by levomepromazine.

Some patients benefit from use of 5-HT antagonists such as ondansetron in bowel obstruction, presumably due to the release of 5-HT from the oedematous gut wall (Twycross & Wilcock). These drugs can be used as an alternative if the above measures fail to control symptoms.

11.2.2.3 Antisecretory agents

Two classes of antisecretory drug are commonly used in malignant bowel obstruction. Firstly anticholinergic drugs such as hyoscine butylbromide, hyoscine hydrobromide, and glycopyrronium block gut receptors and reduce intestinal secretions. These drugs also decrease smooth muscle peristalsis, which relieves intestinal colic. Hyoscine hydrobromide crosses the blood-brain barrier and therefore causes sedation, whilst the other two only act peripherally.

Table 11.1 Drugs used for symptom relief of bowel obstruction and initial dose ranges

Drug		Usual starting dose per 24h
Antiemetics	Metoclopramide	40–80 mg
	Cyclizine	150 mg
	Haloperidol	2–5 mg
	Levomepromazine	6.25–12.5 mg
Antisecretory agents	Hyoscine Hydrobromide	1.2 mg
	Hyoscine Butylbromide	60 mg
	Glycopyrronium	1.2 mg
	Octreotide	250–500 micrograms
	Dexamethasone	6–10 mg

Secondly somatostatin analogues such as octreotide reduce intestinal secretions via a number of different mechanisms. The most important of these is thought to be its anti-vasoactive intestinal peptide (VIP) effects, which is released by ischemic bowel. Evidence suggests this class of drug to be as effective as hyoscine butylbromide in controlling nausea and vomiting, but with a faster onset of action (24 hours versus 72 hours) (Mercedante et al.). Octreotide can be given parenterally by repeated boluses or via continuous infusion and the dose adjusted by effect. This can be in combination with anticholinergic drugs. For clinically stable patients where longer term administration is required monthly or 3-monthly depot injections are available, but as with all somatostatin analogues they are relatively expensive.

11.2.2.4 Steroids

Corticosteroids are sometimes used despite a relatively poor evidence base. Their anti-inflammatory effects reduce bowel oedema and increase salt and water absorption from the gut. In addition they have central antiemetic properties that can work synergistically with other antiemetics. Studies have failed to demonstrate a significant increase in morbidity using dexamethasone at 6–16 mg/day despite theoretical risks of bowel perforation (Feuer & Broadley).

11.2.2.5 Artificial hydration

Whilst the conservative management of an acute or partial bowel obstruction may warrant supplemental IV hydration until the patient is able to tolerate oral fluids once more, for patients unlikely to recover a judgement is made on the risks and benefits of artificial hydration. Potential benefits include the increased levels of hydration contributing to a general feeling of well-being, with reduced levels of confusion in some. Potential burdens include increased intestinal secretions and resultant vomiting, line infection and trauma, decreased mobility and independence and the need for increased healthcare worker input for patients managed in the community. Feelings of thirst (often exacerbated by use of anticho-linergic drugs) are usually more effectively managed with meticulous mouthcare than artificial hydration. For those with well managed symptoms sips of fluid or a liquid low residue diet may be possible if the proximal small bowel is still functioning.

11.3 **Tenesmus, rectal bleeding, and mucus discharge**

Temesmus is the painful sensation of rectal fullness, which is usually caused by local infiltration of a rectal tumour. Symptoms may be exacerbated by smooth muscle spasm or a more constant neuro-pathic pain from lumbosacral plexus infiltration (Rich & Ellershaw).

Primary treatment should be directed against the tumour itself with laser therapy, local resection, chemo- or radiotherapy, but if this is not possible then pharmacological interventions are necessary. Local resection can be achieved by trans-anal debulking either with the urological resectoscope or cryosurgery and there can be some symptom improvement with a defunctioning stoma.

Tenesmus can be resistant to opioid analgesics, so alternative remedies can be used. Smooth muscle spasm can be alleviated by systemic smooth muscle relaxants such as nifedipine or by local application of nitrate based pastes or creams. There are also case reports of botulinum toxin injections to the area to relieve spasm. Neuropathic pain often responds to neuropathic analgesics such as tricyclic antidepressants, gabapentin or steroids. Alternatively a bilateral lumbar sympathectomy is reported to have an 80% success rate in alleviating pain in some centres.

Rectal bleeding can occur as the result of tumour ulceration, following pelvic radiotherapy or from a synchronous pathology. Treatment should be aimed at the underlying cause wherever pos-sible. Rectal bleeding due to a distal colonic or rectal tumour may be amenable to radiotherapy, chemotherapy, embolization via an internal radiologically guided catheter, via endoscopically guided procedures such as laser treatment, cryotherapy or argon plasma coagulation or trans-anal surgery such as cryosurgery or local resec-tion with a resectoscope. Potential management options therefore require a multi-disciplinary approach to ensure the most appropriate treatment is given.

For those patients who are not appropriate for invasive procedures, pharmacological treatments may reduce bleeding and distress. Case reports suggest benefit from use of systemic pro-thrombotic agents such as tranexamic acid in reducing bleeding, or local measures such as application of sucralfate paste to friable tissue.

Suggested reading

Baines MJ, Oliver DJ, Carter RL (1985) Medical management of intestinal obstruction in patients with advanced malignant disease: a clinical and pathological study. *Lancet* **ii**: 990–3.

Feuer D, Broadley K (1999) Systematic review and meta-analysis of corticosteroids for the resolution of malignant bowel obstruction in advanced gynaecological and gastrointestinal cancers. *Annals of Oncology* **10**: 1035–41.

Hulme CW, Wilcox S (2008) Guidelines on the management of bleeding for palliative care patients with cancer. Yorkshire Palliative Medicine Clinical Guidelines Group, accessible via http://www.Palliativedrugs.com.

Matthew R. Dixona, Michael J (2004) Stamosb Strategies for Palliative Care in Advanced Colorectal Cancer. *Dig Surg* **21**: 344–51.

Mercedante S et al. (2000) Comparison of octreotide and hyoscine butylbromide in controlling gastrointestinal symptoms due to malignant inoperable bowel obstruction. *Supportive care in cancer* **8**: 188–191.

Rich A, Ellershaw J. (2000) Tenesmus rectal pain-how is it best managed? *CME Bulletin Palliative Medicine* **2**(2): 41–4.

Twycross R, Wilcock A (eds) (2009) *Symptom Management in Advanced Cancer*. 4th edn. http://www.Palliativedrugs.com.

Chapter 12

New therapeutic avenues in colorectal cancer

Christopher Ramsey, Alan Anthoney, and
Harpreet Wasan

> **Key points**
> - Current research in immunotherapy centres on provoking either a cytotoxic T-cell response or production of tumour specific antibodies
> - Relative success has been achieved with whole tumour cell vaccines. Use of single or multi-tumour derived peptides may be more efficient and cost effective. The results of the 1st randomized trials are awaited
> - Trials in colorectal cancer are awaited for
>   - Autologous dendritic cell vaccines primed with whole tumour cell lysates or tumour derived peptides
>   - Anti-heat shock proteins (HSP) vaccines; HSP are chaperone proteins that present tumour associated antigens (TAA) to antigen presenting cell (APC)s via specific anti-HSP receptors
>   - DNA based vaccines able to deliver low immunogenic TAAs bound to highly immunogenic foreign DNA
>   - Virus vector vaccines that deliver recombinant genes that may express TAAs, co-stimulatory proteins or cytokines that can produce an heightened immune response
> - The liver is the most frequent site of colorectal metastatic disease and organ specific events lead to global loss of quality and quantity of life. Hence organ directed therapy is a rational approach
> - Randomized studies have provided evidence of a survival benefit for one such method, Hepatic arterial (HA) chemotherapy although this has not been broadly adopted
> - Radioembolization consists of administration via the HA of particles loaded with Yittrium 90. Two large scale randomized studies in the first line treatment of liver predominant disease are currently running following provocative data from studies in first, second and third line settings.

12.1 Introduction

This final chapter deals with two areas of contemporary research. Section 12.1 deals with progress in immunotherapy that aims to reactivate the innate immune response against cancerous cells. Section 12.2 outlines the rationale for and methods of organ specific treatment, in the case of colorectal cancer are aimed at controlling metastatic spread to the liver.

12.2 Immunotherapy

12.2.1 Vaccines in the treatment of colorectal cancer

For over a century the response of the immune system to spontaneously arising tumours has stimulated a significant volume of research. In recent years much has been learnt about (a): how certain cancer cells stimulate the immune system resulting in the killing of these cells at a subclinical (immunesurveillance) or, more rarely, an advanced stage (spontaneous tumour regression) and (b): how cancer cells can develop mechanisms that result in evasion of the immune system with subsequent unfettered tumour growth. The ability to stimulate the body's immune system to detect and successfully kill off tumour cells is the clinical goal of the field of tumour immunology. Although naturally immunogenic tumours (melanoma; renal cell carcinoma) have been the main focus for tumour immunologists for many years it has become clear that the approaches to immunotherapy for less immunogenic tumours such as colorectal cancer may be different. There is an increasing body of pre-clinical and clinical evidence suggesting that tumour vaccines may have a role in the treatment of colorectal cancer.

12.2.2 Colorectal cancer tumour vaccines

12.2.2.1 Scientific rationale

The aim of vaccination is to induce or augment an immunological response to a specific antigen (Ag). This immune response is a multistep process that can result in the stimulation of cytotoxic T-lymphocytes or CTL (cellular immune response) and/or production of tumour specific Ab (humoral response).

For an immune response to take place it is of fundamental importance that an antigenic peptide(s) is correctly displayed within the cleft of an MHC molecule on the cell membrane. Class I MHC molecules are found on the surface of nearly every nucleated cell and bind peptides derived from *endogenous* Ag. Class II MHC molecules, however, are only found on the surface of antigen presenting cells (APC), and bind peptides derived from *exogenous* Ag after they have been internalised through phagocytosis or endocytosis and processed in the endocytic pathway.

Tumour cells display certain characteristics that make them more difficult to use as immune stimuli such as reduced or absent expression of MHC receptors and/or co-stimulatory molecules; a high mutation rate allows the development of immune escape mechanisms and the ability to secrete immune-inhibiting factors. On the other hand, the genomic instability of tumour cells together with increased epigenetic modification provides a rich, ongoing source of novel antigens that are potentially immuno-therapeutic targets.

The strategies developed in colorectal cancer anti-tumour vaccination attempt to overcome the functional immunological tolerance of cancer cells whilst taking advantage of the provision of new antigens.

12.2.2.2 Polyvalent vaccines
Whole cell vaccines
Whole cell vaccine strategies use autologous cells (from the patient's own tumour) which thus express the whole range of tumour specific antigens on their surface. To enhance the immunogenicity of the cells the vaccine also includes an immunostimulatory adjuvant.

A Phase III prospective randomized trial of patients following radical resection for stage II and III colorectal cancer used an irradiated whole tumour vaccine with BCG adjuvant (OncoVAX®). Use of the vaccine was associated with specific delayed-type hypersensitivity (DTH) responses to autologous tumour cells and delivered a reduction in risk of disease recurrence at the 5.8 year median follow-up of 22.4%. Overall survival in the OncoVax®-treated group was increased compared with controls, with a relative risk reduction of death of 11.1% and 33.3% in all patients and stage II patients, respectively. At the time of this study neither vaccine or control group received adjuvant chemotherapy as it was not standard of care.

A similar approach using Newcastle-disease virus as an adjuvant along with irradiated autologous tumour cells showed improved overall survival compared to patients receiving surgery alone in a randomized study of 567 stage I–IV colorectal cancer patients. Ex-vivo infection of autologous tumour cells with Newcastle disease virus prior to vaccination, a construct called ATV-NDV, has been shown to increase their immunogenicity. A phase III randomized prospective trial demonstrated that vaccination of colorectal cancer patients with ATV-NDV, following resection of liver metastases, was associated with increased overall and metastasis-free survival.

Dendritic cells (DC) are antigen presenting cells (APC) found throughout the body and can provide an alternative vehicle for vaccine delivery with immune induction. Vaccines can be formed from autologous DC pulsed with allogeneic tumour cell lysates or by chemical fusion of DC and tumour cells (creating fusion cells). Such vaccines can present a spectrum of identified, and as yet unidentified, tumour associated antigens (TAA) on MHC I and II with the result of polyclonal cytotoxic T-lymphocyte induction. Such an approach has shown evidence of activity in other tumour types and although not yet at the stage of clinical trials in colorectal cancer, DC-tumour cell fusions have shown efficacy in murine models.

Heat shock proteins

Heat shock proteins (HSP) are intracellular glycoproteins that constitute the most abundant protein subtype in the living world. They function as peptide chaperones and are transcriptionally upregulated in environments of cellular stress such that peptides are protected and homeostasis maintained. They are known to chaperone TAA-derived peptides from proteosome to endoplasmic reticulum to MHC and present them to DCs via an HSP-specific receptor (CD91). In this way, the need for specific recognition of a TAA by a CTL in inducing a tumour-specific immune response is circumvented.

Following promising results in animal models, the HSP-96-based vaccine, Vitespen® (formerly Oncophage®), was the first autologous cancer vaccine using HSP to be trialed in humans against a number of malignancies including colorectal carcinoma. Induction of CEA- and epithelial cell adhesion molecule (EpCAM)-specific CTL responses was demonstrated in five colorectal cancer patients vaccinated with autologous liver metastasis-derived HSP-96, following metastasis resection. A follow-up study including 29 patients demonstrated that survival was correlated with prognosis (as defined by liver metastasis burden) and specific immune response induction following vaccination.

12.2.2.3 Antigen-specific vaccines

Protein and peptide vaccines

Vaccines composed of specific protein or peptide fragments from TAA of colorectal cancer generally provide a more efficient and cost-effective means for vaccination than whole cell preparations. However single epitope vaccines are often plagued by low immunogenicity.

The two main TAA in colorectal cancer used for such peptide vaccine studies to-date have been CEA (a cell surface glycoprotein involved in cell adhesion) and MUC1 (a membrane-bound, cell-signalling phosphoprotein). Although vaccination studies using recombinant CEA peptide with GM-CSF adjuvant or CEA CAP-1 peptide loaded autologous dendritic cells have shown specific immunological responses (both IgG and CTL) in patients, no large scale clinical trials have been performed to date. Similarly MUC1 peptide vaccines have shown the ability to induce immune responses in transgenic mouse models and patients. Phase III clinical trials of a vaccine incorporating the extracellular core peptide of MUC1 (Stimuvax®) in breast and NSCLC are ongoing but no such large scale clinical trial program of MUC1 peptide vaccines exists in colorectal cancer.

In an attempt to overcome the low immunogenicity of single epitope, vaccines using multiple peptides against different TAA have been developed. Using a novel molecular screening protocol for identifying immunogenic colon cancer specific peptides (from TAA) Immatics Biotechnologies GmBH® (Tubingen, Germany) have developed a multipeptide vaccine for clinical use. A phase II trial in patients with advanced colorectal cancer has used this vaccine as maintenance therapy after standard first line cytotoxic chemotherapy has achieved disease control. The primary end-point of the study is progression free survival (with a comparison against historical controls) and the study has completed recruitment.

Anti-idiotype vaccines

These vaccines are developed by injecting a TAA into a mouse resulting in the production of Ab (Ab1). Subsequent immunization of other mice with Ab1 will generate anti-idiotype Ab against Ab1 (Ab2). Immunization of patients with selected Ab2 (which possess epitopes that mimic the structure of the original TAA) can induce an amplified immune response in the host not only against Ab2 but also for the original TAA.

A vaccine mimicking an epitope of CEA (3H1) was developed in the 1990s and found to stimulate humoral and cellular immune responses in advanced colorectal cancer patients and, given in combination with 5FU, in patients after resection of their primary or metastatic tumour. However, a recent Phase III trial, in which 3H1 was tested in the presence of 5-FU and leucovorin, found no survival benefit vs. placebo when an intention-to-treat analysis was performed. Specific anti-CEA Ab response was, however, correlated with improved survival in both treatment and control arms.

Similarly, a recent phase II trial of colorectal carcinoma patients treated, post-hepatic metastasis resection, with anti-idiotype mAb vaccines to the TAAs, CEA (CeaVac) and human milk fat globule (TriAb), found no overall survival benefit of vaccination plus resection versus resection alone.

DNA vaccines

Foreign DNA is highly immunogenic producing both cellular and humoral immune responses. Within the cell there are a range of molecules designed to detect microbial molecules. These molecules, collectively known as pattern recognition receptors (PRR) can bind to DNA or nucleic acid fragments and stimulate the immune system. This tends to be either through activation of a type 1-interferon pro-inflammatory response or a non-interferon dependent response stimulated through activation of specific cytokines. This ability of foreign

DNA to deliver antigens and engage multiple pathways of immune activation has lead to the development of DNA-based vaccines with the potential to induce strong immunity against weakly immunogenic antigens. In general such vaccines consist of a bacterial DNA plasmid containing a coding sequence of the human TAA of choice under the control of a mammalian gene promoter. Increasingly these vaccines also include coding sequences for proteins that act as immunological adjuvants such as immunogenic fragments of tetanus toxoid. After administration the plasmid is taken up by a range of cells including APC (such as dendritic cells). Using host cell machinery the TAA and immunological adjuvant sequences are translated into peptide fragments that are then presented on the surface of the APC. They can then stimulate the immune system directly.

The route of administration of DNA vaccines has been shown to have a significant influence on their immunogenicity with initial clinical studies. For example the volume of vaccine deliverable by intramuscular injection may not be sufficient to produce an immune response without causing unacceptable local symptoms. Other methods of administration such as electroporation, passing an electric current across the site of injection (skin or muscle) immediately after vaccination, allows greater antigen expression and recruitment of inflammatory cells.

DNA vaccines offer an advantage over other vaccine strategies in that they are much simpler to scale up to mass production than viral vector or cellular vaccine.

To date phase I trials of a number of DNA vaccines have been carried out across a range of cancer types. One such trial including patients with colorectal cancer has used a DNA fusion vaccine combining the sequence of codons 605–613 of the carcinoembryonic antigen (CEA) combined to the tolerance-breaking domain (DOM) sequence of tetanus toxin. This Cancer Research UK sponsored phase I/II study recruited patients who were HLA-A2 positive and whose tumours were known to have expressed CEA (as identified by elevated blood CEA levels). Two groups of patients were recruited - those with advanced tumour with no other standard treatment options (15 patients—12 with colorectal cancer) and another group who had had complete resection of their tumour but were at high risk of relapse (12 patients—6 colorectal). The vaccine was shown to produce robust T-cell responses against both the CEA and DOM fragments and this was more likely in the group of patients without measurable disease. A group of patients (including those without colorectal cancer) developed diarrhoea as a consequence of vaccination and this appeared to be associated with a greater likelihood of falls in serum CEA levels and a longer progression free interval. It has been postulated that the diarrhoea may be an autoimmune reaction related to activity against the CEA fragment. Further studies to confirm this are under development.

The delivery of recombinant genes (expressing, for example, TAAs, co-stimulatory molecules or cytokines) within a viral vector is known to initiate a heightened immune response (that is mainly driven towards the vector proteins), when compared to direct antigen delivery with adjuvant. Following inoculation, viral vectors are able to infect *in situ* DCs and, in doing so, pre-empt a breach in immunological tolerance. Of great importance is the ability of the vector to initiate a response that is optimally balanced in terms of induction of Th subset and regulatory (Tregs, Tr1, Th3) versus proinflammatory mediators.

Poxvirus has been widely investigated as a vector for vaccine delivery, its prototype, vaccinia virus, having been successfully exploited in the eradication of smallpox. It is a double stranded DNA virus able to replicate within infected cell cytoplasm and thus has no ability to integrate into the host genome. Additionally, its large genome permits the introduction of over 10 kb of foreign DNA.

The majority of recent poxvirus vaccine preparations have used a modified vaccinia Ankara (MVA) strain that is highly attenuated having undergone hundreds of passages in chick embryo fibroblasts. A gene that has undergone much research in the context of this vector is that encoding the oncofetal Ag, 5T4, a 420 amino-acid cell-surface glycoprotein expressed on human trophoblast cells and numerous human tumours (80% of colorectal cancers). Following the confirmation of targeted immunity to recombinant MVA-5T4 in murine models, vaccines using this construct (TroVax®) have been evaluated in colorectal cancer patients in phase I and II clinical trials. Initial trials of TroVax® demonstrated a 5T4-specific immunological response (by Ab production or immunoproliferative assay) in 94% of patients. The responses, however, were transient, prompting examination of the vaccine's efficacy in conjunction with chemotherapy. When given in combination with FOLFOX or FOLFIRI regimens, 5T4-specific Ab responses were detected in 91% and 83% of evaluable patients, respectively. ELISPOT assays confirmed peptide-specific CTL responses in both trials and retrospective analyses have confirmed statistically significant inverse relationships between specific Ab and CTL response and disease progression and tumour burden. A phase III trial of the TroVax vaccine was planned in advanced colon cancer but put on hold after a similar trial in renal cell cancer did not achieve its primary efficacy end-point.

Other viral vectors, such as Canary pox (ALVAC) and fowl pox (rF), have been investigated as potential vaccine platforms.

An ongoing challenge to the use of all viral vector vaccines is their induction of neutralizing Ab to viral coat proteins that stymie the efficacy of repeat inoculations. A variety of novel strategies are under development to try and address this problem.

12.2.3 **Conclusion**

As yet no cancer vaccine strategy has produced a therapeutic agent showing sufficient activity against colorectal cancer (either in the adjuvant or advanced setting) to hint of likely progress to clinical usage. However, there remains continued interest in developing vaccines for colon cancer with a wide range of approaches being followed by industry and academic research. This activity, as well as recent successes of vaccines in other tumour types, suggests that this therapeutic approach may still bear fruit as an effective future treatment. It may well be that such vaccines will find their niche in the setting of minimal residual disease with the aim of maintaining remission for prolonged periods of time. The interaction of vaccines and cytotoxic or targeted therapies in colon cancer and the potential roles and sequences of such treatments will be a fertile area for research over coming decades.

12.3 **Organ directed therapy**

The approach of treating metastases with systemic therapies is palliative in intent, whereas surgical resection of limited metastases can be curative (Chapter 9). Unfortunately, less than 5% of all metastatic patients fall into the latter category and the majority of these relapse eventually. The disappointment has been that even with the newer biological agents, the complete response rates and so cure rates from chemotherapy alone remain exceedingly rare. Disease resistance to all agents, on the whole occurs within 1 year. The five year overall survival of all patients with stage IV disease remains at 7% (US SEER, 2009). The challenge is thus to develop treatment pathways that increase the probability of 5 year survival.

The liver is a vital organ and is the most frequent site of colorectal metastases; it leads to organ-specific morbidity, which often translates to dominant global symptoms in terminal care, impacting both quality and quantity of life. Progress in therapies having global impact can thus be organ directed, with rapid advances in medical technologies enabling this. More extraordinarily, focussing on one organ can often achieve better response outcomes that can translate to a bridge to curative outcomes- the ultimate goal of cancer research. Improved outcomes with such a multi-modality approach have already been demonstrated in rectal cancer with radiotherapy and better surgical and imaging technologies. This section will focus on the liver as a specific target of organ directed therapeutic approaches. In principle, however other metastatic sites such as lung and peritoneum are developing similar paradigms.

12.3.1 Chemotherapy and liver specific-outcomes

Response rates to systemic chemotherapy over the last 20 years have been gradually improving, as new active agents developed, but the proportional gains in terms of overall survival benefits and per-centage of complete responders have been disappointing. However, Liver-specific response rates have major relevance, if advantage can be taken with other interventional modalities at the time of maximum chemotherapy response. This has been retrospectively and compara-tively demonstrated in many phase III trials. Traditionally the other modality has been liver surgery, but other non-operative modalities are increasingly being used, expanding the possible patient cohorts and selection criteria. Biologically, this has rational as residual disease post-chemotherapy will contain resistant populations that other modalities eradicate (i.e. potentially eliminate the putative cancer stem cells).

There is good evidence from clinical trials that:

1. A synergistic approach with systemic chemotherapy and liver surgery in *operable* liver metastases (1–4 deposits), can improve disease free survival outcomes
2. In a subset of patients, chemotherapy can downstage *inoperable* liver metastases enabling potentially curative surgery with similar outcomes to *operable* liver metastases
3. Liver-directed chemotherapy infused via the portal vein (PVi) or Hepatic artery (HAi) improves overall survival. A meta-analysis of six HAi trials has shown benefit in terms of increased response rates as compared to the equivalent systemic chemotherapy and improved statistically significant overall survival advantage (14.5 versus 10.1 months $p = 0.0009$). However, many centres have methodological and practical problems with HA or PV infusion, making it less popular as other developments occurred. The evidence base does still prove the principle of potential benefits of organ directed strategies
4. Synergistic approach with systemic chemotherapy and palliative liver ablative techniques such as Radiofrequency ablation (RFA), traditionally considered non-curative, can improve disease-free survival outcomes.

Thus, there is good clinical evidence that liver focussed approaches, in a multimodal context can significantly and incrementally benefit selected patients. Research in the technologies, delivery, poten-tial synergies and multi-modal integration is rapidly offering new possibilities.

12.3.2 Selection of local versus loco-regional modalities

Despite rapid imaging advances, the best cross-sectional technolo-gies (CT and MRI) have a maximum liver resolution in the order of millimetres. This equates to approximately 10^7 cancer cells, which even with functional imaging such as PET, only improves by one order of magnitude at best. Thus retrospective analysis of the timing and patterns of relapse observed after attempted curative resections of colorectal liver metastases can define the non-visible micro-metastatic disease burden probability for each situation, allowing the development of suitable patient selection criteria. The information from the EORTC Intergroup 40983 randomized controlled Phase III trial is the unbiased benchmark (gold-standard) in the best prognostic groups. It demonstrates that in the presence of 1–4 visible potentially curable metastases at presentation, 50% or more of patients will have relapsed within 18 months of curative liver surgery, many within the liver. By three years only one quarter to one third of patients remain disease free. Thus, by definition the majority of patients (approx. 70%) have 'invisible' micro-metastatic disease, even when selected for curative surgery with less than 4 liver metastases. This data highlights that the major strategic approach to curing liver confined metastases should be whole organ-directed (local and regional) versus imaging-directed (local) approaches. Alternatively, it confirms that the majority of patients will need a multi-modal sequenced approach with other systemic or loco-regional strategies.

12.3.3 **Local liver therapies (Table 12.1)**

These are image-guided based approaches and an extension of liver surgical approaches. They aim to eradicate any visible metastases at the time of staging and attempt to do this via non-surgical or per-cutaneous means. The aim is to reduce the morbidity of the liver surgery, i.e. without open surgery, reduce hospital stay (improve recovery and quality of life) and at the same time potentially allowing repetitive and multiple interventions to eradicate visible metastases. They can also increase the time that patients are off cytotoxic chemotherapy, especially if are used to consolidate an initial response. They are not liver restricted and can target lesions in the lung, adrenal, skin and even bone. The main limitation is that that by definition they cannot target non-radiologically visible lesions (i.e. 5 mm or less or micro-metastases). Furthermore, the real evidence of benefit to patients in terms of randomized control trials are lacking with quality of life and morbidity outcomes poorly documented. They also often have the same restrictions of liver surgery in terms of the anatomy and amount of functional liver reserve that must remain. Nevertheless, with good patient selection, some patients do benefit. On the contrary, patients with progressive chemoresistant disease that is non-chemotherapy responsive, rarely benefit.

12.3.4 **Loco-regional liver therapies: whole organ based approaches (Table 12.1)**

These are non-image guided or whole-organ based approaches and a natural extension of the HAi and PVi chemotherapy approaches

Table 12.1 Non-surgical, non-systemic approaches and technologies currently in clinical use for organ-confined liver-targeted treatments. Whole organ approaches have a major advantage of theoretically targeting micro-metastatic (non-imaging visible) disease, but can frequently be super-selective also (segmental or lobar)

Therapeutic Approach	Interventional	Whole Organ	Limitations	Comments
1) Organ directed Chemotherapy				-No clear advantages over systemic chemotherapy -not all agents can be given in this way
Hepatic arterial infusion (HAI)	Yes	Yes	-Indwelling infusors -thrombosis -increased liver toxicity -non-patient friendly	
Portal venous infusion (HAI)				
2) Organ directed Chemotherapy combining particle embolization to tumour	Yes - As above but chemotherapy pre-loaded on particles	Yes - Potentially Introduces regional selectivity also	-Hepatic abscesses -Severe Pain on administration -post embolic syndrome prolonging hospital stay	Embolization causing tumour ischemia not-evidence based in CRC -as in (1) above
Debiri (Irinotecan pre-loaded)				
Bead Block™ (pre-loaded beads with Doxorubicn)				No evidence that all drugs have CRC effect if given this way
3) Conformal External Beam Radiotherapy	No	No	-Volume of treatment limited by whole organ tolerance of Radiotherapy doses (see text)	-can be combined with systemic chemotherapy -not limited to organ can target lymph nodes for example if image visible
IMRT/IGRT				
Cyberknife				

(Continued)

Table 12.1 (Contd.)

Therapeutic Approach	Interventional	Whole Organ	Limitations	Comments
4) Internal Radiotherapy/ Brachytherapy delivered via Hepatic artery: SIRT Y^{90} Radioembolisation preloaded on resin or glass particles	Yes	Yes -but particles allow regional super-selectivity for local or lobar approaches	-Dose limited by whole organ tolerance of Radiotherapy doses (see text) otherwise RILD -Complex logistics -Leakage of particles to non-target organs	-Phase II/III data combined with systemic chemotherapy demonstrates highest response rates recorded
5a) Local ablative technologies -dependent on extreme temperature changes for tumour cell kill	Yes	No	-treating lesions > 4 cm have significant morbidity including hepatic abscesses	-Percutaneous radiologically guided -patient friendly -can be done intra-operatively also combined with major liver resections
Radiofrequency ablation (RFA)				
Microwave ablation				-Faster process than RFA
Cryoablation			-vascular fracture	Being superseded

5b) Local ablative technologies -dependent on Ultrasonic technology for cell kill	Both approaches available	No	-Hepatic abscess	-Clinical outcomes evidence base lacking in CRC -Theoretically synergistic with chemotherapy as cell membranes sonicate potentially opening up membrane channels
High intensity focussed ultrasound (HIFU)	No			
Irreversible electroporation (IRE; also called Ultrasound Nanoknife)	Yes		New technology appears non-heat dependant	As above -evidence suggests pro-apoptotic without inducing significant heat or necrosis -less effect on vasculature and fibrous tissues may be a significant advantage

IMRT: Intensity modulated radiotherapy; IGRT: Image-guided radiation therapy; RILD: radiation induced liver disease as the liver has a dual blood supply. They are based on the principle that liver tumours including metastases obtain their cancer neo-vasculature predominately through the Hepatic artery (70–85% of blood flow) whereas the portal vein supplies the majority of normal (non-cancerous liver parenchyma). This creates an 'Achilles heel' that can be potentially clinically exploited.

Loco-regional therapies aim to eradicate metastases *irrespective* of whether they can be visualised by imaging techniques, on the basis that the majority of patients have micro-metastases and thus the majority are not selected for local or surgical liver approaches. They therefore expand the cohorts of patients that are suitable for additional interventions, although are currently considered non-curative.

These approaches are liver restricted and may not be transposable to other organs due to anatomical, physiological or safety constraints. The specific benefit to patients in terms of randomized control trials are on-going, with the most advanced clinical trials data available from hepatic arterial radio-embolization.

12.3.5 Liver radiotherapy, Hepatic arterial radio-embolization (RE), Selective internal radiotherapy (SIRT brachytherapy) with Ytrium-90

Chemoradiotherapy is an integral component of the multidisciplinary approach for the management of localized rectal cancer. However, a key limitation of external beam radiation in the treatment of liver tumors is the tolerance of normal liver parenchyma to doses higher than 35 Gy, which is unfortunately below that required to eradicate most tumours (for mCRC this is estimated at >70Gy for monotherapy or >50Gy with concurrent chemotherapy as a radiosensitizer). Hence, the concept of a more targeted vascular approach using radioembolization (also termed selective internal radiation therapy, or SIRT) began to develop over 50 years ago. Technical problems hindered the adoption of this approach until the development of the current generation of products now in use for over 15 years. Both resin and glass microspheres containing Yttrium-90 (^{90}Y) as the therapeutic isotope are used. The resin microspheres (SIR-Spheres^{TM}) have the largest clinical evidence database in CRC (at least 30 trials reported to date). These have shown that radioembolization using ^{90}Y microspheres is associated with high response rates in the first line setting (>80% in combination with systemic 5FU and oxaliplatin), randomized studies have suggested a survival benefit beyond first line chemotherapy and reported series have shown activity in chemo-refractory ('salvage') patients. The quantitative benefits appear to be greatest when this intervention is used earlier in the colorectal treatment paradigm as well as in combination with concurrent chemotherapy. Two pivotal adequately powered randomized phase III controlled trials

(FOXFIRE and SIRFLOX) are examining the role of ^{90}Y resin microspheres in combination with chemotherapy for the first-line treatment of colorectal hepatic metastases. In salvage, where no other treatment options remain there is compelling data that significant palliative benefits can be achieved in 1/3 of patients selected for liver-predominant metastases, with good performance and liver functional status. The short-term toxicities appear manageable with the most serious ones being a 1–3% risk of radiation hepatitis and 2–5% risk of a radiation gastroduodenal ulcer, which are self limiting in most cases. Little is known about the long term effects on the liver parenchyma which will be tested in the ongoing trials.

12.3.6 **Summary**

Advances in systemic chemotherapy have improved non-curative, median-survivals incrementally in metastatic disease over the last 20 years. However, to effect higher cure rates (survival >5 years and above), there remains dependency on selection for liver surgical excision of residual metastases, as the complete pathological response rates of chemotherapy alone remain imperceptible. The keys are thus to have improved patient (clinical) and molecular selection, combined with expanding the populations suitable for integrated combination modalities including liver surgery, leading to complete eradication of organ confined metastases. Rapid technology developments with reducing morbidities make this a current reality, providing that a significant evidence base follows from concurrent clinical trials, to make informed decisions about safety, efficacy and quality of life, for better long-term qualitative and quantitative outcomes. There is increasing evidence that these multitude of technologies can be synergistic as opposed to additive, if selected and tested properly. The application of an innovative multidisciplinary approach that integrates advanced approaches (such as radioembolization and local ablative therapies) should ultimately allow the benefits of curative hepatic resection to be extended to a broader group of patients.

There may also be significant quantitative palliative benefits, hitherto ignored, if the concept of 'Vital organ' salvage develops an evidence base. That is targeting metastases early in the treatment pathway in specific organs such as the liver, may have an overall higher impact on the patient than generally controlling systemic metastatic disease in other sites.

In the future multidisciplinary approaches will be truly cross-speciality in *effect*, with integrated treatment options discussed on a regular basis from the outset. Not, as is currently often the case, being single- technology or speciality dependent, or at the salvage (end) of the treatment pathway, when unfortunately, no realistic treatment options exist and the patient cohorts are significantly smaller and less functionally able.

Suggested reading

Adam A and Mueller P (eds) (2009) *Interventional Radiological Treatment of Liver Tumours*. Cambridge University Press.

Fioretti, D; Iurescia, S; Fazio, VM; Rinaldi, M (2010) DNA vaccines: developing new strategies against cancer. *Journal of Biomedicine and Biotechnology*. Epub.

Harrop R, Drury N, Shingler W, et al. (2007) Vaccination of colorectal cancer patients with modified vaccinia ankara encoding the tumor antigen 5T4 (TroVax) given alongside chemotherapy induces potent immune responses. *Clin Cancer Res* **13**(15 Pt 1): 4487–94.

Merika E, Saif MW, Katz A, Syrigos C, Morse M (2010) Review. Colon cancer vaccines: an update. *In Vivo* **24**(5): 607–28.

Meta-analysis group (1996) Reappraisal of hepatic arterial infusion in the treatment of nonresectable liver metastases from colorectal cancer. *J Natl Cancer Inst* **88**(5): 252–81.

Morse M, Langer L, Starodub A, Hobeika A, Clay T, Lyerly HK (2007) Current immunotherapeutic strategies in colon cancer. *Surg Oncol Clin N Am* **16**(4): 873–900.

Nordlinger et al. (2008) Perioperative chemotherapy with FOLFOX4 and surgery versus surgery alone for resectable liver metastases from colorectal cancer (EORTC Intergroup trial 40983): a randomised controlled trial. *Lancet* **371**(9617): 1007–16.

Schreiber, TH; Raez, L; Rosenblatt, JD; Podack, ER (2010) Tumor immunogenicity and responsiveness to cancer vaccine therapy: The state of the art. *Seminars in Immunology* **22**: 105–12.

Sharma RA, Van Hazel GA, Morgan B, et al. (2007) Radioembolization of liver metastases from colorectal cancer using yttrium-90 microspheres with concomitant systemic oxaliplatin, fluorouracil, and leucovorin chemotherapy. *J Clin Oncol* **25**: 1099–1106.

van Hazel GA, Pavlakis N, Goldstein D et al. (2009) Treatment of 5-fluourouracil-refractory patients with liver metastases from colorectal cancer using yttrium 90 resin microspheres plus concomitant systemic irinotecan chemotherapy. *J Clin Oncol* **27**: 4089–95.

Wasan H, Kennedy A, Coldwell D, Sangro B, Salem R (2011) Integrating Radioembolization With Chemotherapy in the Treatment Paradigm for Unresectable Colorectal Liver Metastases. *Am J Clin Oncol* PMID: 21278562.

Index